SACRED CEREMONY
FOR A
SACRED EARTH

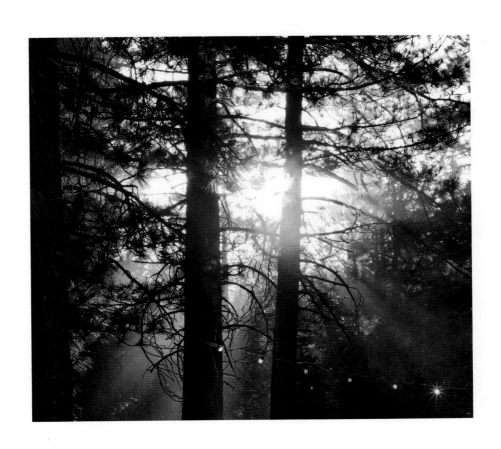

Quarto.com

© 2025 Quarto Publishing Group USA Inc.
Text © 2025 Aniwa Digital
Photography © 2025 Aniwa Digital

First Published in 2025 by Fair Winds Press, an imprint of The Quarto Group,
100 Cummings Center, Suite 265-D, Beverly, MA 01915, USA.
T (978) 282-9590 F (978) 283-2742

Fair Winds Press titles are also available at discount for retail, wholesale, promotional, and bulk purchase. For details, contact the Special Sales Manager by email at specialsales@quarto.com or by mail at The Quarto Group, Attn: Special Sales Manager, 100 Cummings Center, Suite 265-D, Beverly, MA 01915, USA.

29 28 27 26 25   1 2 3 4 5

ISBN: 978-0-7603-9212-6

Digital edition published in 2025
eISBN: 978-0-7603-9213-3

Library of Congress Cataloging-in-Publication Data available.

Design: Landers Miller Design
Cover Image: Elizabeth Gottwald
Photography: @AwakenChannel: Pages 12–13, 14 (top), 29, 105; Audrey Lane: Page 110; Ben Geo: Page 224; Bryan Mir: Pages 6, 153, 200 (bottom); Chris Dodds: Pages 61, 215; Daniel Garcia: Pages 11, 23, 64, 97, 99, 115, 124 (top), 131, 197, 200 (top); Elizabeth Gottwald: Pages 5 (#8), 32, 35, 93, 179; Erin Donalson: Pages 1, 21, 95, 119, 124 (bottom left); Ivan Sawyer Garcia: Pages 106, 186; Jethro Tanner: Pages 8, 26, 41, 50, 53, 55, 68, 73, 100, 109, 188, 203, 210; Katya Castillo: Pages 103, 120, 208; Kelly Daniels: Pages 16, 19, 162; Marc Baptiste: Pages 4 (#6), 5 (#11), 14 (bottom left), 45 (left), 46–47, 49 (top), 79 (bottom right), 124 (bottom right), 141 (bottom left); Marcia Machado: Pages 5 (#13), 14 (bottom right), 127, 207; Matua: Pages 49 (bottom left), 49 (bottom right), 164, 167, 168; Nana Ixquik: Pages 79 (top right), 80; Papali'i: Page 204; Raine Skye: Pages 4 (#2), 63, 66–67, 82, 85, 129 (right), 133, 141 (bottom right); Safaa Kagan: Pages 31, 42, 70, 90, 134, 135, 144, 218; Shutterstock: Page 56; Ursula Vari: Pages 4 (#3 & 4), 5 (#10), 24, 38, 45 (right), 77, 116, 129 (left), 137, 138, 141 (top), 142, 149, 151, 157, 161, 170, 177
Illustration: Chiffon Lark, Chiffon Lark with consultation by Eugene Baatsoslanii Joe on page 22, and Tata Mario on page 181

Printed in China

Indigenous Wisdom for Healing and Transformation

SACRED CEREMONY
FOR A
SACRED EARTH

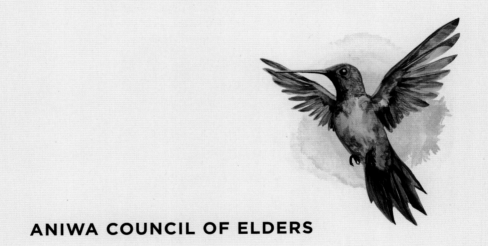

ANIWA COUNCIL OF ELDERS

FAIR WINDS

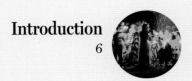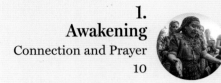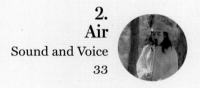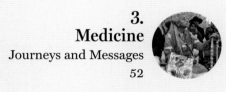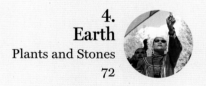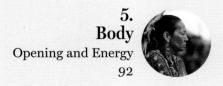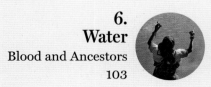
CONT

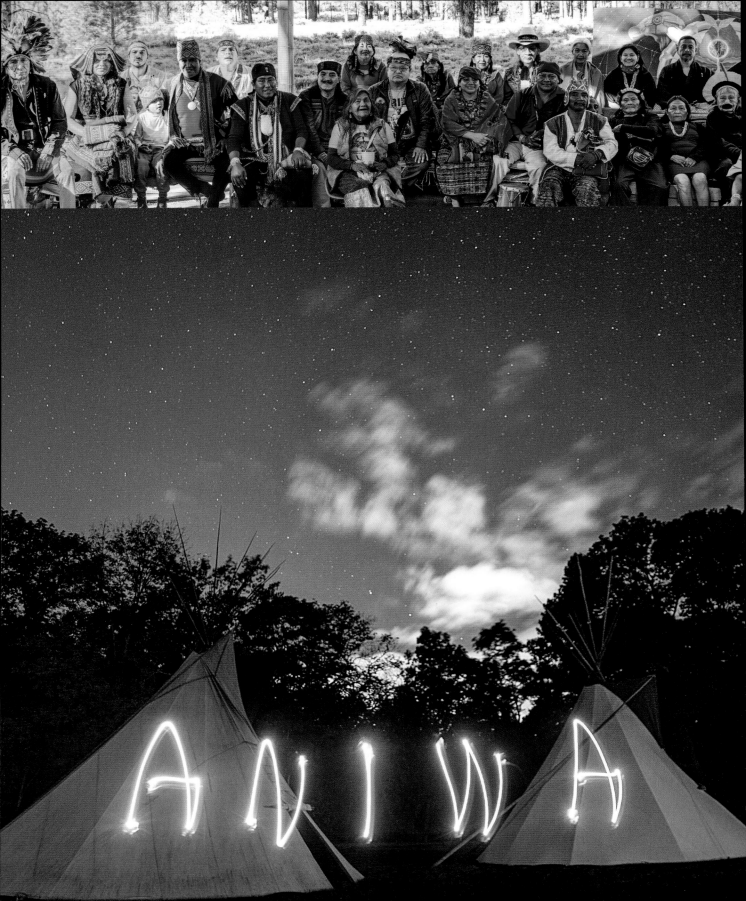

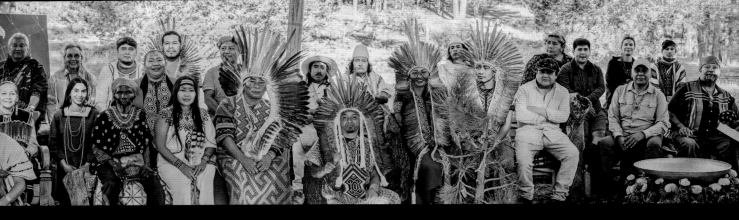

Introduction

Aniwa is a prayer that manifested in 2017 as an annual gathering, retreats, an online platform, and now a ceremony book, bringing together cultures and wisdom to amplify the voices of Indigenous elders worldwide, sharing their teachings, stories, ceremonies, and healing practices. Aniwa embodies a vision of unity, inviting us to transcend cultural divides and embrace our shared humanity.

These ancestral cultures are the original stewards of timeless wisdom and have long coexisted in harmonious relationships with the Earth, recognizing a sacred reciprocity at the heart of all existence. In their ontology, we are all children of Mother Earth, destined to return to her embrace, our bodies composed of her elements, our spirits intertwined with the cosmic dance. However, the march of modernity has caused a fundamental disconnection from these foundational truths, leading to myriad societal maladies: mental health and health crises, isolation, racism, loss of cultural identity, overconsumption, misinformation and distrust, and environmental degradation that, ultimately, stem from the same root—human disconnection from the sanctity of life, nature, and the divine.

Aniwa emerges as a direct response, a guiding light beckoning humanity back to ancestral wisdom, restoring the forgotten bonds with nature and self. It calls upon us to awaken our ancestral lineage, to rekindle the flame of connection with our roots and the natural world.

Through the ancient wisdom of the elders, we embark on a journey of self-discovery, unveiling the purpose of our souls and reclaiming our intrinsic relationship with Mother Earth. Across the world, our collective well-being is intrinsically linked to the health of our planet. Aniwa invites us to embrace sacred reciprocity, acknowledging our responsibility to nurture Mother Earth as she nurtures us and to give back in balance with what we take. Through sacred ceremonies and offerings, we release emotional, mental, spiritual, and physical burdens, opening our hearts to receive the abundance of life's blessings. In healing ourselves, we heal the planet, honoring the interconnectedness of the web of life.

The Aniwa Gathering stands as a testament to this transformative vision, a sanctuary where a plethora of different cultures converge in reverence for life. Elders and leaders from around the world impart their wisdom throughout the Gathering, igniting the flame of remembrance within each participant. Through ceremonies, songs, and dances, we realign with the rhythms of nature, reawakening to our sacred duty as stewards of the Earth. In this communal space, we reimagine a world guided by spirit where every action reflects harmony, reverence, and gratitude.

The profound experiences shared through these gatherings and initiatives have culminated in the creation of this book, a vessel to preserve and transmit the teachings of these Indigenous elders, ensuring their wisdom continues to inspire future generations to walk the path of unity and Earth stewardship.

As we navigate the challenges of the present age, the wisdom of the Aniwa elders in these pages offers a guiding light, illuminating a path of beauty and balance. Ancient prophecies speak of a time of renewal where humanity awakens to its interconnectedness and embraces a new paradigm of living. Aniwa invites us to fulfill these prophecies by co-creating a world rooted in reciprocity, compassion, and reverence for all life, inspiring individuals to embody the change they wish to see in the world.

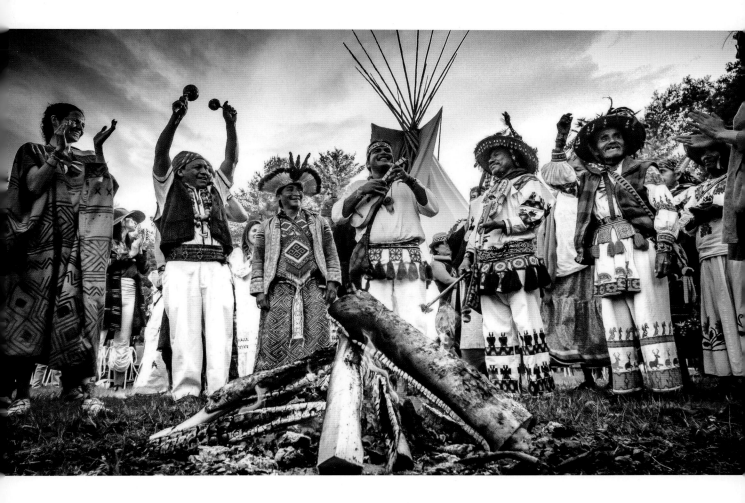

Through our sister nonprofit organization, the Huya Aniwa Foundation, we practice active reciprocity by raising funds for cultural preservation, land back efforts, food sovereignty, and environmental initiatives, supporting Indigenous communities to sustain their traditions and continue to thrive on their ancestral lands.

Through the wisdom of elders and the power of community, we reclaim our place as guardians of Mother Earth, stewards of a future guided by love and respect for all life. May we join in the spirit of Aniwa, honoring the sacred web of all life and weaving a future guided by harmony for generations to come.

—Vivien Vilela, Aniwa Founder

Awakening
Connection
and Prayer

✳

Awakening is being conscious of the spiritual, emotional, mental, and physical experience with an attitude of gratitude. Hear from Aniwa's elders about how they open their eyes and how they start their day. Find in their words ways to connect with nature and activate your spirit with each new beginning every moment brings. This moment marks the beginning of this book's journey, but, as in the cycles of nature, it also marks a place to return again and again and again as a reminder to remember to awaken.

Notice what and how the elders speak about awakening through connection and prayer.

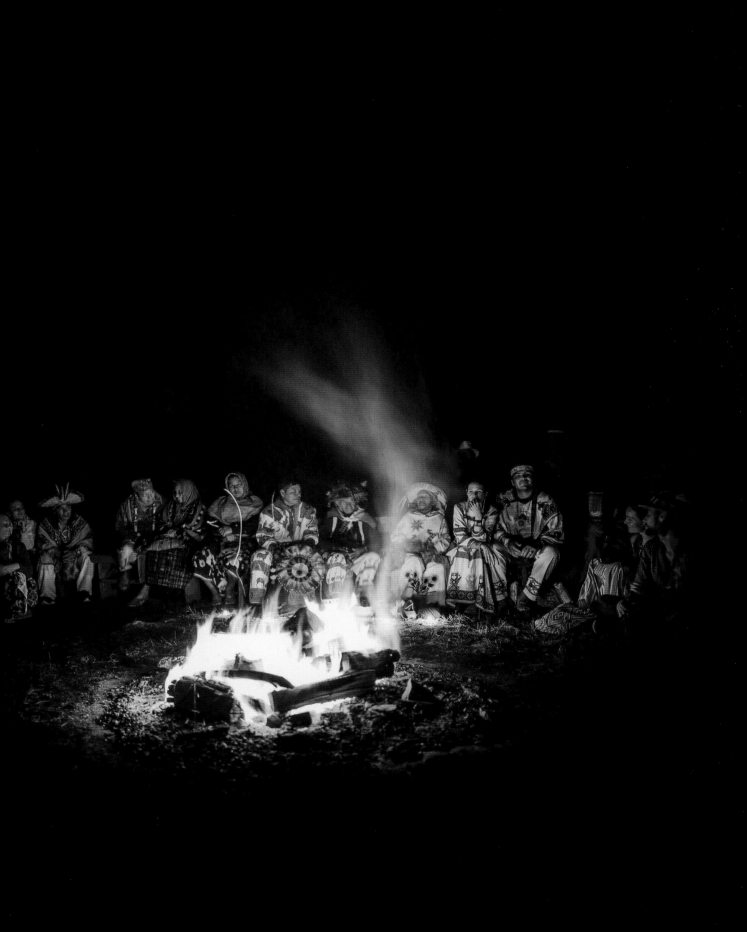

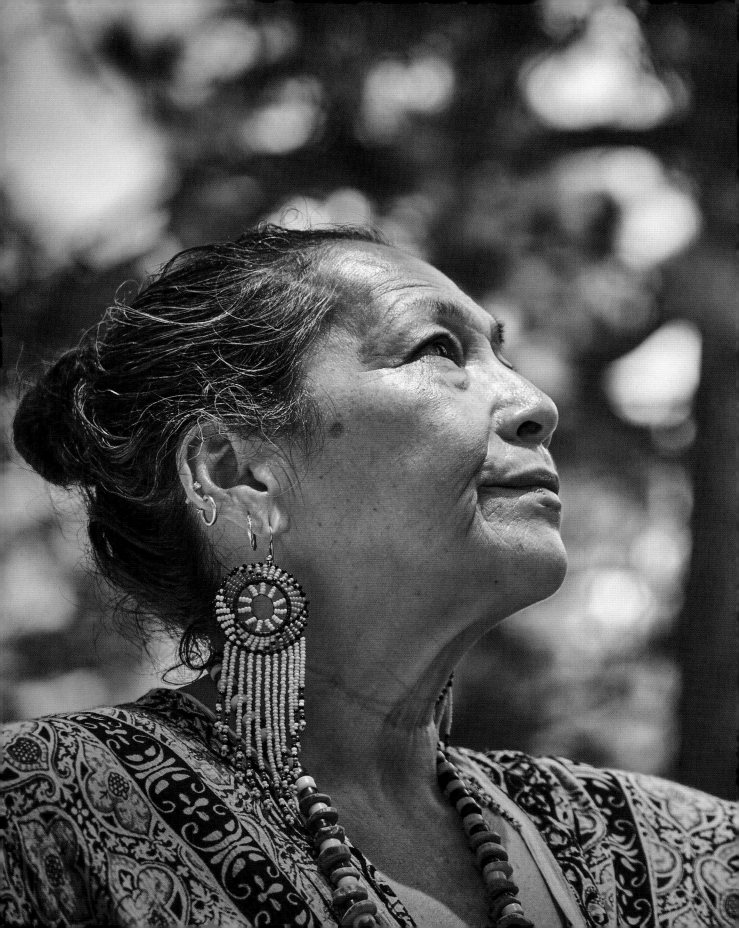

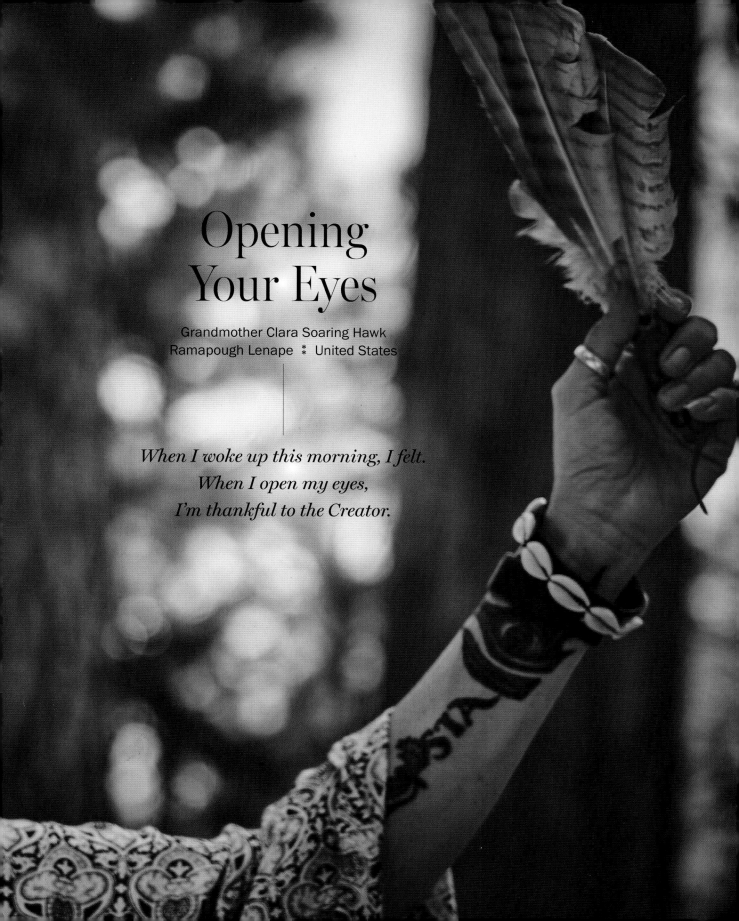

Opening Your Eyes

Grandmother Clara Soaring Hawk
Ramapough Lenape ✳ United States

When I woke up this morning, I felt.
When I open my eyes,
I'm thankful to the Creator.

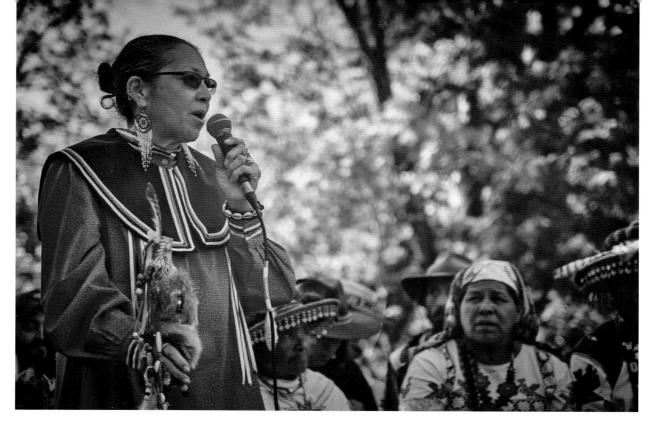

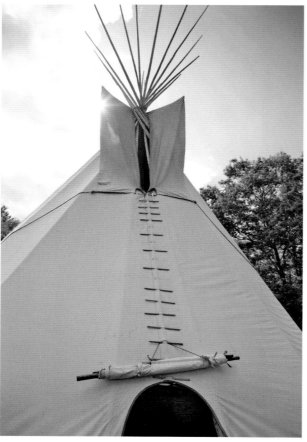

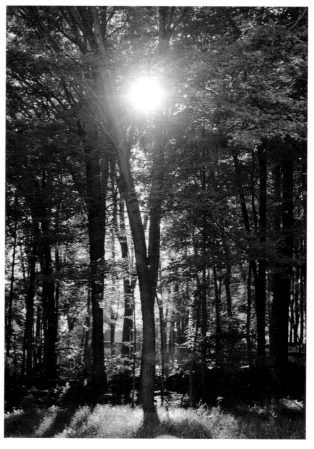

I'm thankful to the Creator for allowing me to be in my right mind, clear-headed, to have use of my limbs, and to be able to go forward having the chance to serve in a good way—another chance to make things right. I am thankful and I am prayerful that my children and grandchildren are in this same fashion.

This morning, I felt such a pull to the land. I have developed a living, viable, tangible relationship with so many ancestors who once journeyed here. I have developed a relationship with the trees, the land herself, the water. I believe with my whole heart that we serve a greater purpose in this world for healing and for teaching and for bringing people together who would probably never have met. Even if they live so close, they are in a place so far from each other.

For me to be in this position has heightened every sensibility that I have spiritually. It has awakened me and shown me how to appreciate and to walk in this way of ceremony. I have a pact with the land. Whenever I have any negative issues in this natural world, I travel the distance to the land and I bring all that I have to her. She will then relieve me of my problems and I sing, drum, and pray her my thanks.

The premise is that I leave my ego and my mind behind me when I come forth through those gates. This allows me to absorb and not be afraid of all that exists in the woods. I am most comfortable sleeping outdoors hearing the sounds of the birds and the animals, hearing the water, and listening to the voice of the trees. My spirit is always on the land—always seeking to be near nature.

I don't know if you've ever heard a lake waking up after a winter's sleep. When staying at a cabin, while throwing wood in the fire, I heard the birds having a conversation with the lake. It's so incredible to hear the lake wake up. It sounds like a cannon going off. You just stand there and wait, knowing that it's going to reach you. With anticipation, you wait . . . and then it happens! You hear the big boom and you feel that reverberation under your feet. It is so powerful.

Always, I state my intention when I come to the land. I put down tobacco and ask permission to come forward. I have never gone forward until I've been beckoned by the leaves. It's like a tunnel of wind blowing down the path and all the leaves are fluttering to say, "Come . . . come forward now." It is so beautiful. It happens every time.

I have a relationship with the land to move forward in a good way, believing in reciprocity the way the Creator has shown me. It is possible to see the spirit world visually and to communicate through a form of energy. The answers I receive are given through a transference of energy. It's something that I have learned to trust.

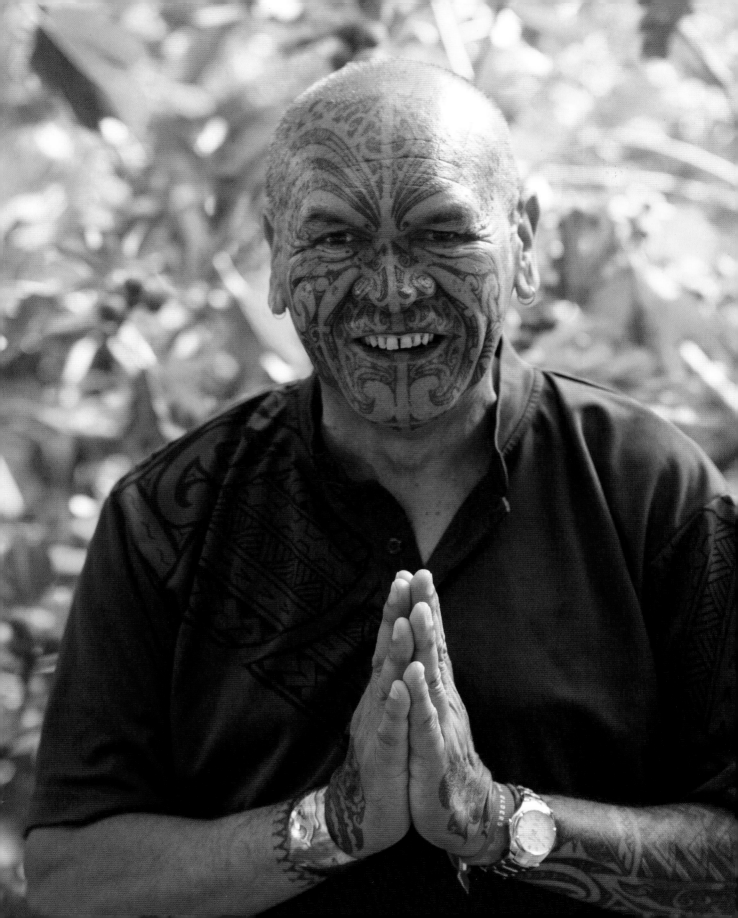

This Prayer That I Offer

Louis Te Kouorehua Kereopa (Matua)
Māori ✳ New Zealand

I am sharing with you.

It has to be pure. It has to be clear.

When you talk to someone, like a tree, you talk straight to the tree. You don't go around the tree because by the time you return to the front of the tree, you're told your story will be changed.

I have a Māori prayer. It is for the guidance and protection of the many readers of this book as a simple message of Love and Gratitude. Through this book, it will touch the hearts of many.

This prayer came to me in a quiet moment. It's a well-known prayer that I said quite regularly when I used to teach the ceremonies. My whole life, I never knew that my work and my whole teaching was actually a ceremony! In the humility of my heart, I didn't want to have that kind of star over my head, but I laugh just to know that my journey on this planet Earth was to be of service. I gave my youth to beloved God and to all our ancestors before coming to live this lifetime knowing that it will continue, as we all do for many lifetimes, the lesson that brings peace to the karma that surrounds us. Being eternal beings, it will fulfill itself in its own time for each of us. We are here as individual beings and are all special. Our spirits are forever. It's like a river that flows. That's our spiritual journey. It's endless. It keeps going on and on forever. I know that one day, it may be many lifetimes, we will always cross each other's paths.

Prayer Extract

He honore, he kororia ki te Atua
Honor and glory to God . . .

He maungarongo ki te whenua
Peace on Earth

He whakaaro pai ki nga tangata katoa
Good will to all people

Hanga e te Atua, he ngakau hou
Develop a new heart

Ki roto, ki tena ki tena o matou
Inside all of us

Whakatongia tou Wairua Tapu
Instill in us your sacred spirit

Hei awhina
Help us

Hei tohutohu i a matou
Guide us

I nga mahi mahi mo tenei wa
We need to learn today

Haumi. . .eee
Join
Hui eee
Gather

Taiki eee
Unite

Tihe mauri ora eee
Tis the sneeze of life

------·-------

Note: In Māori culture, the sneeze of life refers to the mucous coming from a baby's nose as the first breath of life. Hupe, or snot, represents the first breath to unblock the nose; it is represented in Māori carvings. That sneeze indicates the blessing of the Holy Spirit who breathes life into all creation.

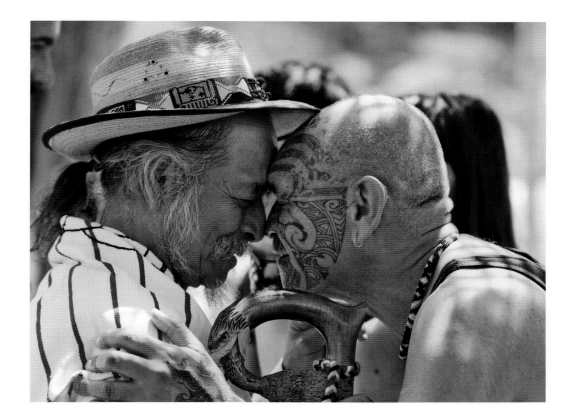

There are so many people out there searching for an answer on how to connect, how to connect with the Creator and with themselves. You don't have to rely on any prayer of any language at all. It's you and me. We are the Creator. We are that temple. We are that vessel to talk to your mother and father, to the Earth, because it's all the Creator. You can talk to the sky. You can talk to the birds. You can talk to the insects. It's so tremendous how powerful the love of the Creator is everywhere and in everything.

Ask, *How am I feeling?*

It has to be your own words. That's where the power is, because you're you. We are beings beyond our understanding. Just be yourself. You are not a separate being at all. We are not separate in a separate room. There is no line. No. We are one family and we will always be one family.

Prayer is about talking. The word "pray" actually belongs in a Christian sense, but "prayer," for us, is more. It is the law of nature. The law of nature is where we are and what we are a part of. We are that law. We are that breathing and living law of life . . . of nature.

My prayers begin with the first breath I take when I wake up. My prayer begins every day. We are a living prayer of creation. We are the light. We are the continuous light that shines in the world of the manifest, of the Creator. Everything we do, everything we say, everything we experience is a part of that. It's a love that's beyond love itself.

Beyond, beyond, beyond and will always be beyond.

We will forever be on that eternal journey.

Staying Connected with This Earth

Patrick Scott
Diné (Navajo) ✳ United States

There's quite a bit of activity that goes on up in the universe that we don't know anything about.

There are very few things we know about the darknesses that exists out in the universe and those play major roles in who we are. In the morning time, when that darkness lifts, the light comes in. In that light is the dawn, the early dawn spirit. The spirits that come are two deities, the Haalch'eyalt'i (First Talking God) and Haalch'eghaan (Second Talking God) are the Gods of Wisdom. So, when we grow up, as young Diné people, we are told to go run in the morning, and yell as you run. By doing this, those Gods learn to recognize your voice. So, when you sing and pray, they will be able to recognize your voice and fulfill your songs and prayers. As Diné people, we believe these Gods carry wisdom and teach us in ways that you build communications with. These prayers and songs replenish us as our days start.

This is the "Earth Song" and prayers; we have twelve words for twelve major deities that we see and that we name when we sing the "Earth Song." When doing Hozhooji (justice and harmony) ceremonies, these songs honor the Earth we walk on and live on. All living beings live on this Earth, so these are the songs and prayers for the place we live, the Earth.

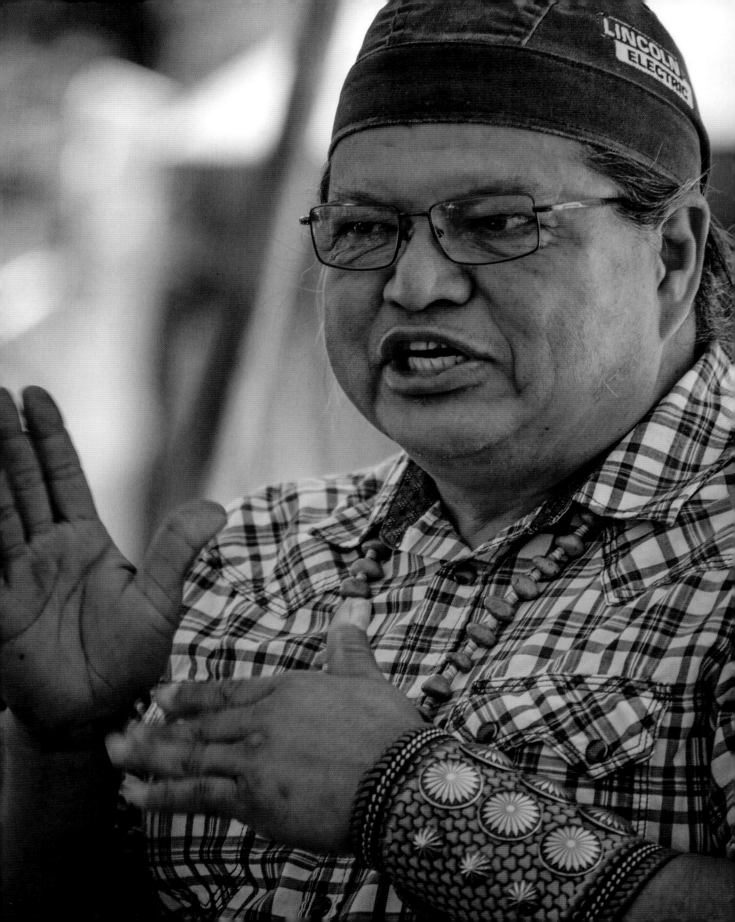

The "Earth Song" and prayer is to call out to these twelve deities:

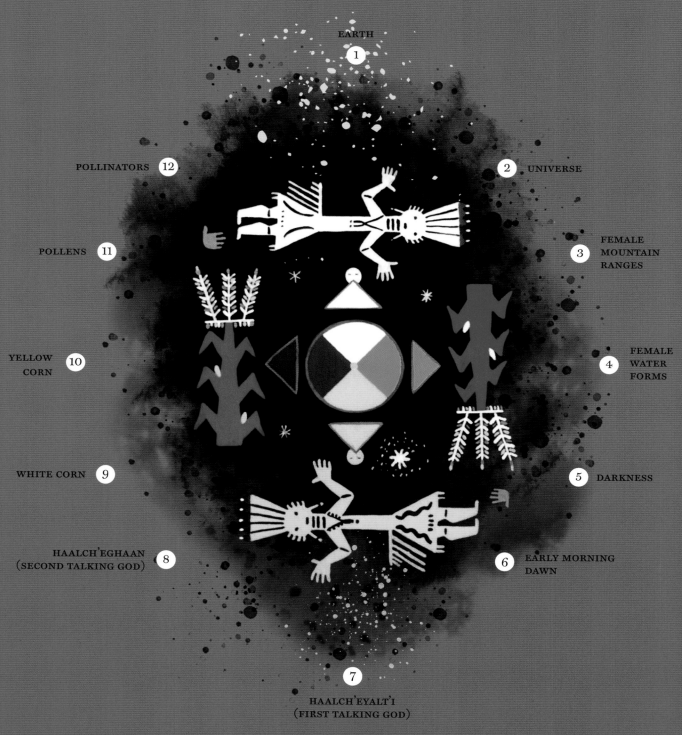

EARTH
1

POLLINATORS 12

2 UNIVERSE

FEMALE
3 MOUNTAIN
RANGES

POLLENS 11

FEMALE
4 WATER
FORMS

YELLOW 10
CORN

WHITE CORN 9

5 DARKNESS

HAALCH'EGHAAN 8
(SECOND TALKING GOD)

6 EARLY MORNING
DAWN

7

HAALCH'EYALT'I
(FIRST TALKING GOD)

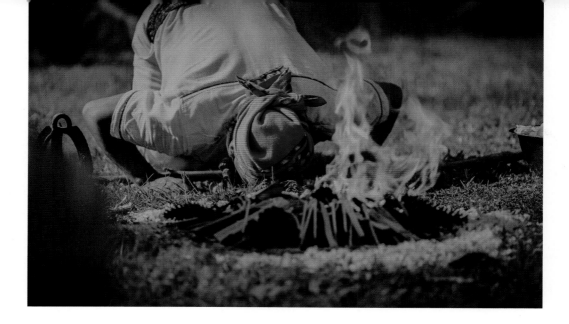

When you want to connect to the Earth, start walking on the Earth. Old Diné ways, we believe that when our body is in contact with this Earth, that is where connections are built. When we disconnect, like walking on pavement, walking with shoes, and sitting on chairs, the disconnect starts happening. When your bare feet feel the Earth or when you take off your clothes and sit on the sand, that's where it comes into your body. It's basic bacteria for your immune system. That was the way it's supposed to be. Then, modern society put socks and shoes on us. They covered us, and now there's a lot of disconnect happening. All the bacteria that are supposed to be in our bodies are being distorted. All over the world, you see it. People are disconnected. It's all distorted. Very distorted.

It's off balance everywhere. I travel quite a bit to different places and see the same thing over and over.

Every week, we go into the sweat lodge when we are close to home. When we go into the sweat lodge, we take off our clothes and then we sit on the Earth. After we leave the sweat lodge, we sit on the ground and put sand on our body. We take some sand and we put it on our body. Then, we sit and let it dry on us. Afterward, we brush it off. All the dry skin, it comes off with the sand—it kind of sands it off. Then, all the pores of your body are open. When you put the sand on your body, it replenishes the nutrients or the bacteria that are supposed to exist on our bodies. They penetrate. That's how you replenish a lot of your gut system, the major immune system and the bacteria that exist there. That's a very common practice. We do this all the time.

From there, we sing all kinds of protection songs. The "Earth Songs." These are the major grounding, starting songs—the ones that move everything for us. The Earth and the sand are really medicine for us. When you get into the Western ways of thinking, you get into jobs and you get into all these money-making things and you forget. You forget about all the things that nature provides for you. It gets distorted. That's where a lot of people all over get disconnected. We just get into the motion of jobs and the daily things that we do, but then we forget we're on this Earth.

We live on this Earth. We sleep, we walk on this Earth. Everything we do is on this Earth. That's part of being the animal that we are. We cannot disconnect from that part.

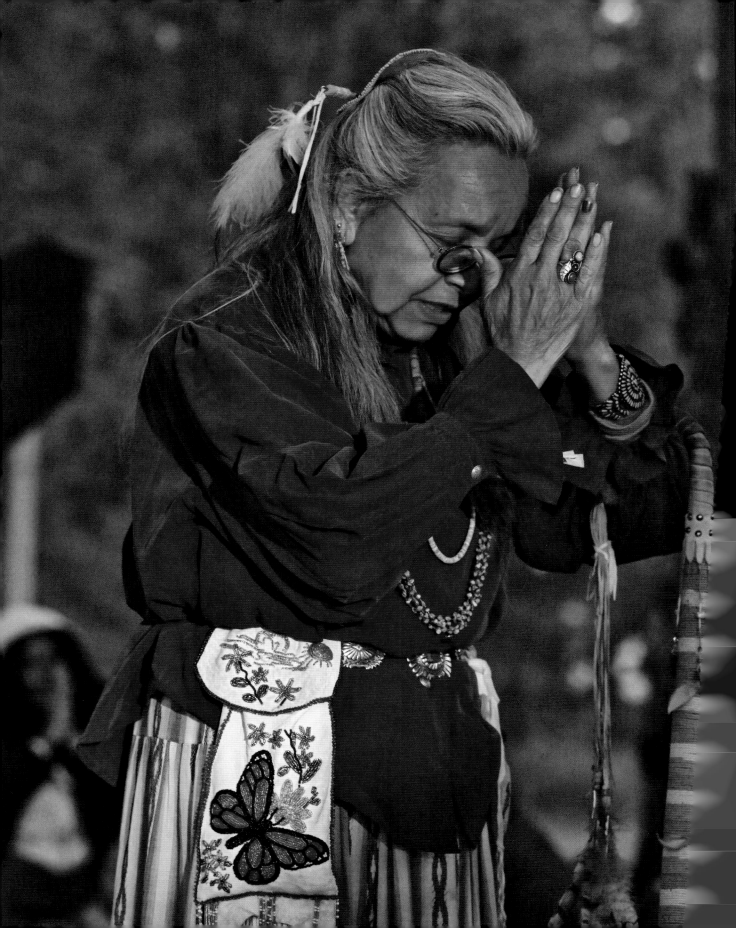

Creating a Relationship with Hom Eh, Our Sacred Earth Mother

Grandmother LánéSaán Moonwalker
Yoeme and Apache ⁎ United States

I want to send my love and greetings
to all of you from my heart of hearts.

I wish to share with you what it is to have an intimate, sacred relationship with Hom Eh, our sacred Earth Mother right below our feet. Part of the reason for sharing this is because, when you are not raised with that being an essential part of living, inclusive of conception and death, it is extremely difficult to build into your beingness later. It is a part of your being whole and at one with the greater whole.

I would like to translate what "Hom Eh" means. These words mean "our shared Mother." The understanding is this is true for everything that walks the Earth, that flies in the sky, that slithers on her, that swims in her waters and sets their roots in her. Everything that is living. We perceive that rocks, shells, the sand, the air or the wind, and the soil that make up her surface body are also living. All of us are her children, and she is our shared Mother.

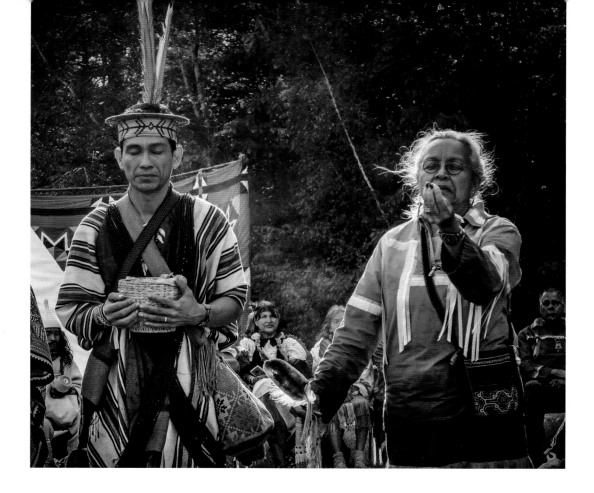

The Practice

Acknowledge your biological parents for having given you life. Acknowledge that they brought you into the world. They, too, are part of her children regardless of how much they were involved with her or not. If you identify as full or part Indigenous from around the world, you may be lacking in a full or solid connection with her. Actually, we are all Indigenous to Earth Mother. In the modern world, it is good to consistently reconnect with her every day and throughout the day.

After acknowledging your parents for having brought you into the world, take the time to acknowledge her, Hom Eh. We literally can experience her in a visceral, bodily way when we are fully bonded to her on an electromagnetic level. It is not in our heads. It is not in the ethereal psychic realm. It is a bodily experience.

This is not done by sitting in a room, separated. Ideally, you go outside to put your feet and hands directly on her and greet her from your heart of hearts as your Mother. Go to your heart center. Contemplate all the ways, all the times you have been moved by her and the natural world. For us, the most sacred time that one does this process is at sunrise and sunset when she and our day star, Father Sun (known to us as She'a Huelo), are in intimate connection from our perspective as humans. Think of some of those sunrises, those sunsets that have been meaningful. Perhaps earlier today you heard a bird singing. Perhaps you have seen the first or the last of the leaves coming out as the seasons change. It is from this place of heart connection that you would do this practice.

The Ceremony

✻ Contemplate all the ways, all the times you have been moved by the natural world.

✻ Put these in your heart center. Convert them into a pool of light and energy. Then, with all of your beingness—your body, your emotions, your mind, your eternal essence—create this pool of life force energy made of all that you love that is natural (such as flowers, animals, trees, the ocean, or sun). It is good to imagine a tinge of golden light to it to make sure you are connecting through your eternal essence. It may include a full rainbow or a few select colors.

✻ Send this energy through your arms and your hands to her as you humbly, gently touch her.

✻ Send it through your feet or knees, or through any part of you that is in contact with her. If you are sitting upon her, send it through your whole rear.

✻ The next place you send this energy from is what is globally referred to as your third eye. We refer to this as our mind's eye: our center of connection and communication.

✻ Send this loving energy as a rainbow and offer it. Do not demand of her to exchange with you. This offering is a gift of your gratitude and love and respect. When you give in this way, particularly through your hands and your feet, it goes directly to her.

✻ You may also offer through your breath on the outtake. The Divine-Sacred-Energies-That-Move-All are constantly sharing with us through our breath. That includes her. Make your gift offering and ask that she would receive this.

✻ In receiving her exchange back with you, be patient. Wait. It will come.

Your intention here is that you have a sacred commitment with her as Hom Eh. This is where you sleep, where you walk, where you make love. This is where you are born and where you die. For all that time, each and every time we go out and walk upon her, we do this with intention that it is done with gentleness and humility.

We greet her in our first step out into the morning. We greet her on our last step coming inside at the end of our day. You will learn as she returns to you her love, respect, help, and support that this is what true unconditional love is. Allow this life-breath of love in as you breathe; let this saturate you throughout. And on the next outtake of your breath, send back to her another burst of gently loving appreciation. Be in true gratitude. Be in true love.

In a gentle, loving way as one of her children, acknowledge her formally and ask her to re-embrace you.

It's just out of habit and our modern culture that we have become divorced from her. This is extremely important every time you take a sacred walk in nature, every time you do gardening, each and every time you sit directly on her in prayer. Be with her when you are having a picnic, or any time you are laughing and giggling with your favorite dog, cat, tree, person, time of day.

It is with deep gratitude that I have had this opportunity to talk to all of you. I hope that you start this practice. It's important to do 7 minutes. Why 7 minutes? Seven is a very sacred number. Part of that is because there are the four directions around us. The fifth is the one below to Hom Eh; the sixth is above to She'a Huelo. The seventh is here at our heart of hearts, the center of our beingness. We have seven visible planets. There are seven visible stars that make up the Big Bear and the Pleiades. For a lot of Indigenous Peoples, the Yoeme and Apache included, seven is the most sacred number.

You're fighting against your laziness. Welcome to being human. That's our nature. Don't take this personally. These are just the facts of how we are.

We have inertia here also, so there's a bigger principle at hand, a bigger law that we have to put extra effort in getting these energies moving. Thus, the process takes 7 minutes minimum. You may work a little harder if you want. Do 14. You are better off doing 7 minutes daily or twice daily than spending a whole hour doing this meditation once a week or every once in a while, when you think about it. Consistency is the most important thing.

I send you my love and prayers. I hope you take my words to heart and do your practices. From my beingness to yours: Shi'deh. We are whole. We are complete. The circle is one.

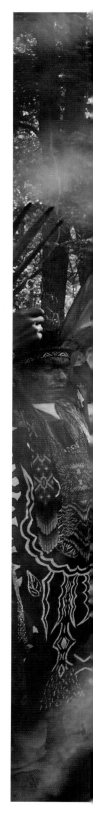

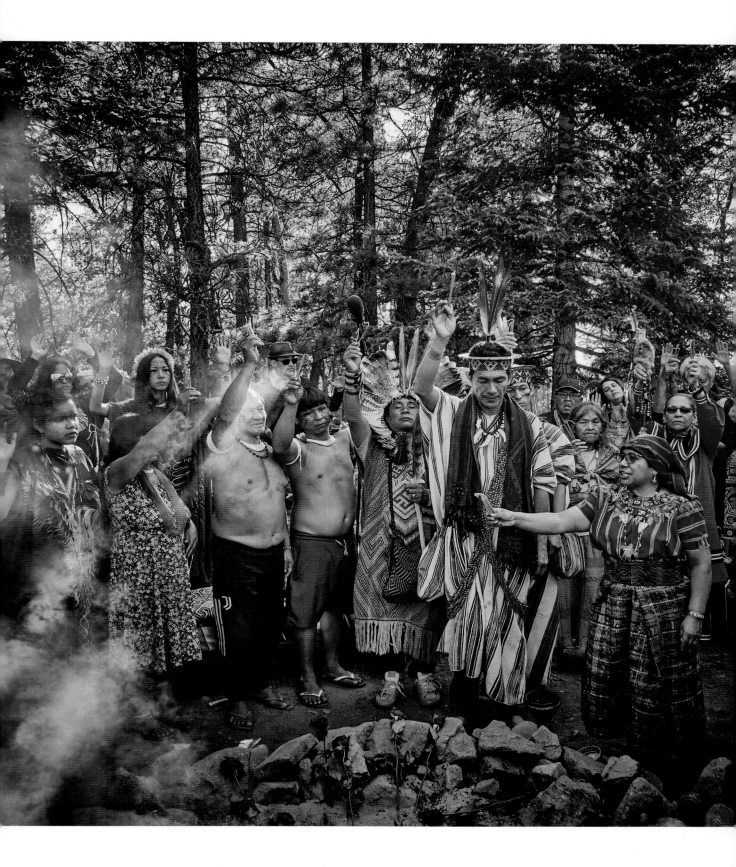

TWILA CASSADORE

Apache ✣ United States

Twila Cassadore (San Carlos Apache Tribe) has been working with San Carlos Apache, White Mountain Apache, and Yavapi peoples for the past 25 years, addressing health and social issues. She works on a number of community and cultural preservation projects reconnecting the local youths with their ancestors' way of life and diet. She is also a professional caterer. Twila is the founder and face of the grassroots organization Native Mothers Against Meth and is featured in the Netflix documentary *Gather*, which explores the fight to revitalize native foodways.

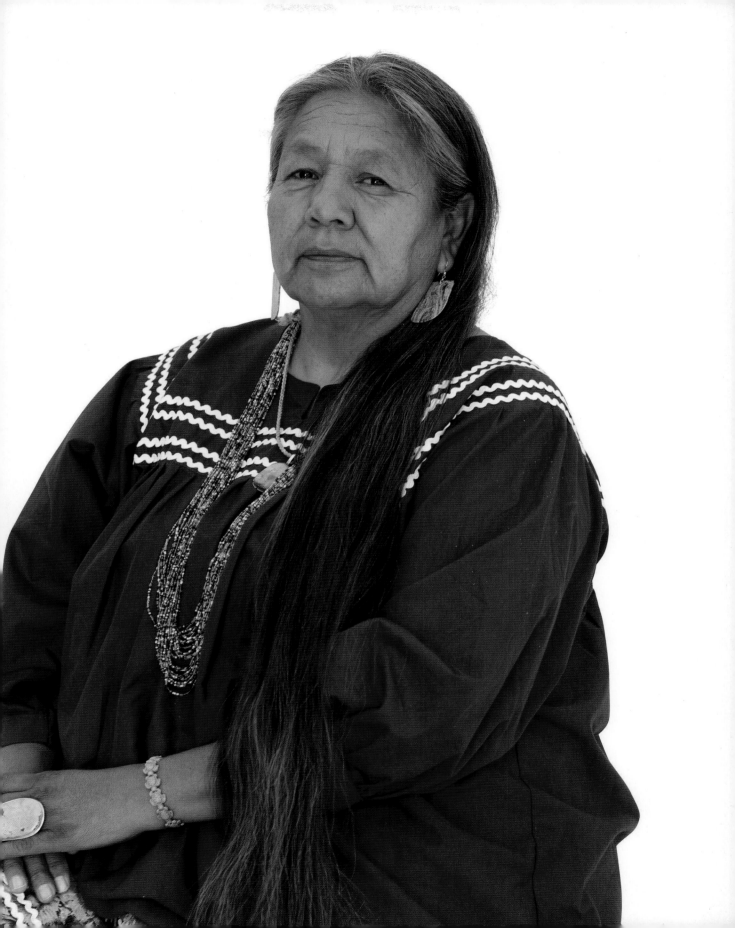

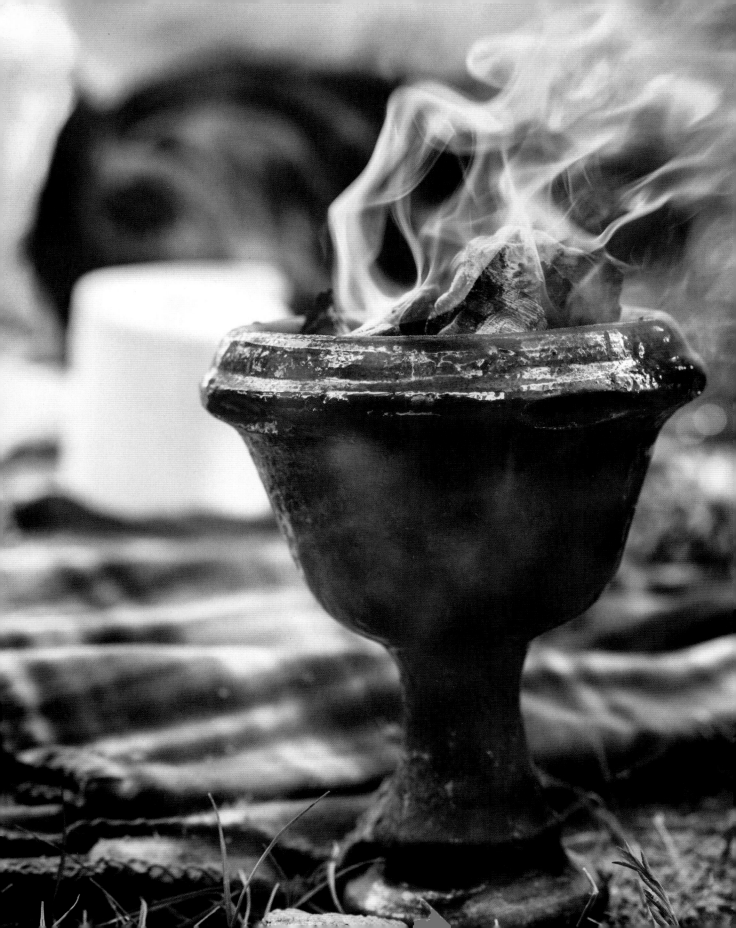

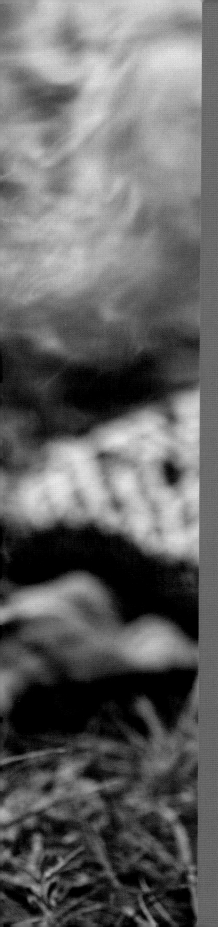

Air

Sound and Voice

✳

Air is what moves. Through wind and voice, air carries the vibrations of beingness in the breath of life shared by people, planet, and all that lives in between. Hear from our elders about how they breathe, how they speak, and how they carry vibration.

———

Notice what and how the elders speak about air through sound and voice.

How to Work with Stones to Release Stress, Grief, and Negative Energy

Twila Cassadore
Apache ⁑ United States

She does hear our footprints when we walk on her.

She does hear our heartbeats.

She does hear our prayers.

She's never seen color,
but she's always heard us as we walk on her.

That's why we have to be kind to her;
to be gentle and pray for each other.

It's not about color, it's not about race,
it's not about anything of that nature.

We all live on Mother Earth.

We all have to help take care of her and try to live in this balance.

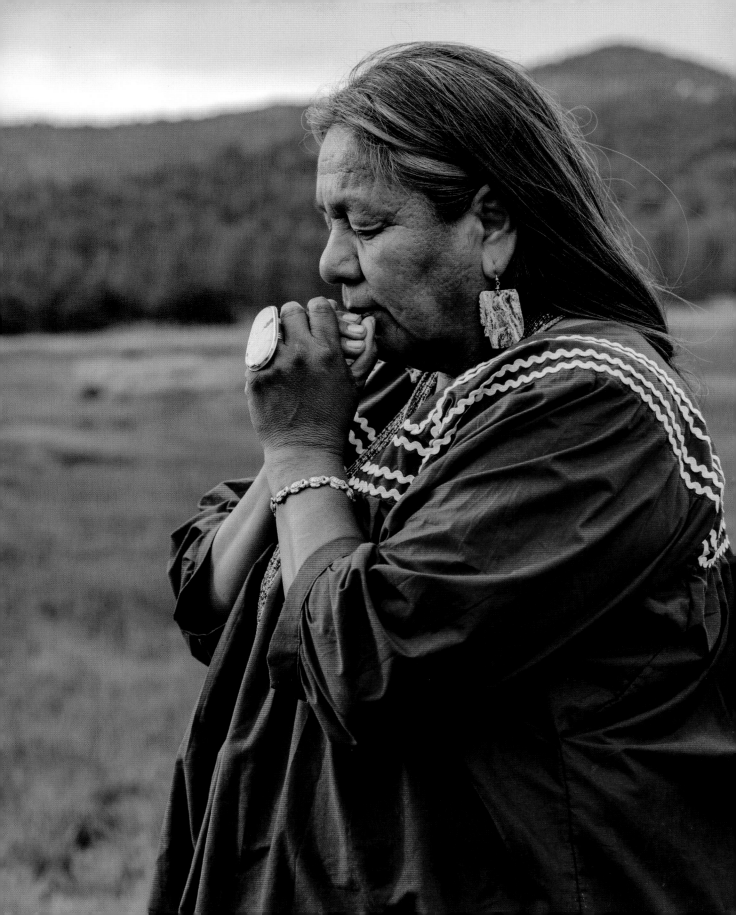

If you close your eyes and listen, the sound of people gathering and sharing sounds like rain. It sounds like rain dancing. That's the beauty of when people gather. It's in the energy we all bring without knowing how powerful those energies are.

I'm going to share a little of myself and how I began my journey.

My journey is very hard. It wasn't simple to get where I'm at. I'm very thankful for where I am today. I've been lost in this life for a lot of years. I grew up outside of the community in a very self-sustaining family. We planted our food, we foraged it, we hunted it. We killed our own beef. We did everything that people would say is not normal. I would go to school with my foraged food and some people were not nice. It was a complete culture shock for me. I'd never been around anyone else but my family.

Through time, I got disconnected from that life. I truly loved of foraging, harvesting, of hunting the rabbits, the quails, the doves, squirrels, and all these different animals. It was a happy life. That changed when peopled looked at me like, "Oh you're so poor, you cannot buy your food." That became a mentality that colonization developed and imposed upon many, many native tribes and indigenous people; that we are poor because we did not buy, did not have electricity, because we hauled our water. That was the most beautiful time in life. It caused a lot of heartbreak for me growing up as I got lost through time.

I had to go to the stones. I had to go back and reflect on what happened to me in life in order to heal. The elders, they took me out one day when I was in my lost mind. We went to go collect willows for the baskets and materials we were going to use for traditional ceremonies. They took me to the river where something happened to me.

As we were collecting, they let me wander out into the river. I don't go to the river. I don't swim. I've never swum. I've been scared. I've been on beautiful waters all across this country, but I've never gone in them. I just walk along the side. I'm scared of water. It's just a fear that's still part of my life. They took me out there, and as I walked through the water, I cried. My elders knew what they were doing. I could smell the dirt. I could smell the willow. All these senses came back to me from that point in time. I cried because I let the pain go. I could carry this pain no more. I cried because I found myself in the midst of love of Mother Earth. The wind blew on me. The birds were around. The sun rose and shined on me. I've never felt so loved in my entire life until that day when we picked the stones.

In our educational system, we are never taught how to heal. We are taught how to be successful. We are never taught when to let go, how long to grieve. We are never taught how to be happy. There is nothing about happiness in our education system. We have to teach ourselves that. We have to find people that help us with that part. I share this knowledge with my community and with young people that dealt with things similar to the many hard things I went through.

The Practice

- Find a stone. Whatever stone you want.

- This stone is something you can carry with you, with your family, with your loved ones.

- You come to it with anxiety, with anger, with resentment about things that happen at home and in culture.

- Take the stone, close your eyes, and blow on the stone.

- Put the stone close to your heart.

- You're going to close your eyes and imagine.

- Think about the most beautiful place you've been where you've seen water. You're going to put yourself there.

- Where you see that river, you're going to put your right foot forward just a little because you're going to be touching the water in your mind.

- Stand there and just let the water flow on your feet.

- In your heart, if you're grieving someone, you're going to see them on the other side of that river standing in a beautiful place.

- Then, you're going to tell them you love them.

- If it's not today, maybe another day; but for those of you that are ready to let go, let them know it's time.

- Tell them, "I'm going to let you go and travel on."

- Tell them you love them again and put your feet back.

- Blow on the stone.

- When you are ready, walk down to a field and place the stone.

Take as long as you need. If you need to sit a while, stay a while. It's a time to cry. It's a time to let go. We're never taught when to let go, but what I'm sharing with you today is for you to carry for your family, for your loved ones, your community, where you work. This is something for you to share. We walk with Mother Earth and she shares her love with us every step we take, even with the smallest stones.

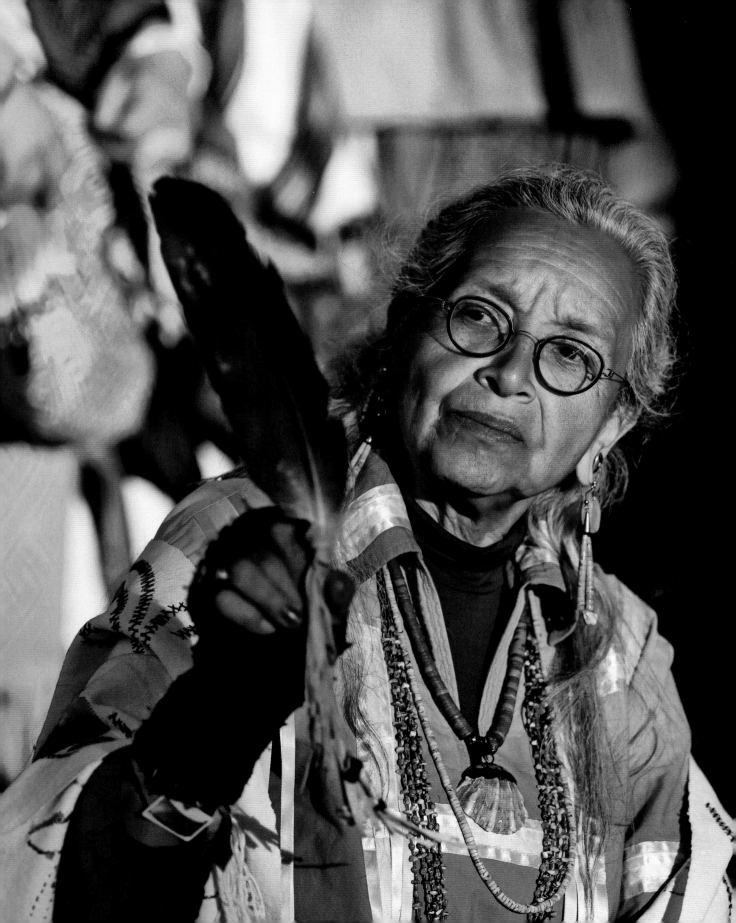

Breath of Beingness

Grandmother LánéSaán Moonwalker
Yoeme and Apache ⁑ United States

Greetings to all of you
from my heart of hearts to yours.

I want to share with you about sacred breath.

Almost every single spiritual and religious group acknowledges that our breath is one of the most important things for us to be able to engage with. Many Indigenous groups feel that it is one of the primary foundational pieces that is important for us to be conscious of, aware of, and to use as a form of meditation and prayer. I would like to share a practice with you.

The invitation is to close your eyes. Just be with your breath. Listen to your breath. If your mind wanders or your emotions wander, thank them very much and return to listening to your breath.

CLICK HERE TO SEE GRANDMOTHER LÁNÉSAÁN MOONWALKER DEMONSTRATE THIS PRACTICE.

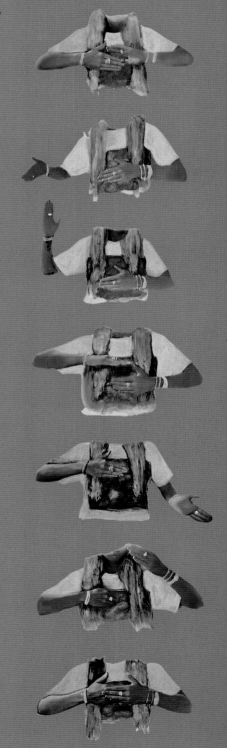

✴ With the first breath, I would like you to bring your thoughts, your emotions, your beingness, out of the past and into the now. We do that with the hand movement—taking our left hand and bringing it to our heart center.

✴ On the next breath, bring your consciousness that is in the future to the now. We do that with a sweep of the right hand, which is about the future, and bring it to our heart center.

✴ With your next breath, give thanks to your body, your beingness, for this breath. Be aware of it. Allow it to become gentler and slower.

✴ With the next breath, give thanks and gratitude. Give thanks to the air around you, which is the blanket surrounding our beloved shared Mother, Hom Eh. Give thanks for its blessing of beingness and being a part of this exchange.

✴ With the next breath, breathe in the blanket of nurturance and support you share with all of Hom Eh's children, whether they have feathers or four legs or fins that swim in the waters. Give thanks if they are elements, rocks, and All-That-Is.

✴ With the next breath, give thanks to this life-giving blanket of air. This is the breath of sacred beingness.

✴ With the next breath, on the exhale, send out your love and gratitude to all around you, All-That-Is. Understand that you are sharing back with the greater whole your love and gratitude as a part of the greater whole.

✴ With the next breath in, as this energy comes and nurtures you, the Energies-and-Power-That-Moves-All is breathing you. They breathe you and you breathe them. Engage with this exchange. This is why we call the ultimate creative principle of the whole "Sha'sha Pu'yeh." The translation is, "As I breathe, so am I breathed." Each moment, each breath, you have this opportunity to be in alignment and whole with the All.

✴ It is the flow of a figure eight, and it is within the circle of your whole beingness. When we do this, we have our left palm open and the back of our right hand on top of it, with both palms facing toward us, oftentimes in our lap so we are also in the sacred circle of life and death and of beingness and a part of the whole. With each breath, you have the opportunity to breathe and be breathed by the sacred powers that move all throughout all time. All space. Now and always.

✴ We are whole. The circle is complete. We are as one, with love and gratitude.

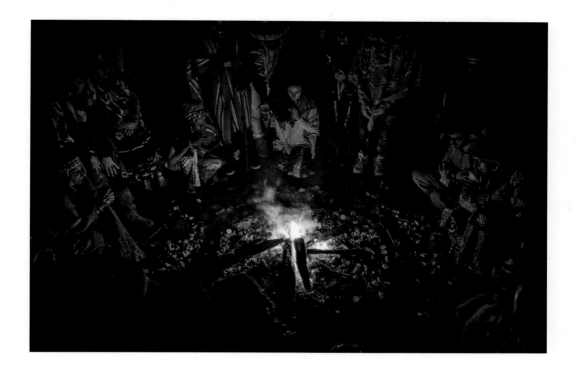

We as Indigenous People are naturalists through observation and awareness. We became aware through our breath that air is a carrier because we didn't ever cut off our psychic sensory system of sound and vibration and ethereal colors. We became aware through our breath that the plants are exchanging their breath with us. Science in today's world has finally caught up with Indigenous Peoples and understands this exchange. We provide carbon dioxide, which the plants need to be able to process and create sugars, and thus live. We need oxygen and a few other components to do the same thing, to live and metabolize what we are taking in, such as water.

Like many Indigenous Peoples, we understand that all the elements have a spirit, a life. When I refer to the air, the atmosphere, as a blanket, it is because we perceive and understand that the movement through the winds is Earth Mother's breath. Of course, the air and the atmosphere will be here much longer than you and I will, but many billions of years ago it was not around Earth Mother—and she was not here yet either. Everything in the universe, everything lives. In that, it has a spirit. This movement is how our thoughts and prayers are carried into the greater whole.

We emphasize when working at this process that it is done in a prayerful place of gratitude and love. Because when we're angry and expressing it, that also gets carried by the wind and affects all around us. Then, it comes back to us. When we express a blessed and loving energy through our breath, all is nurtured and supported, including ourselves.

I hope that this will help you understand the aliveness of everything that is.

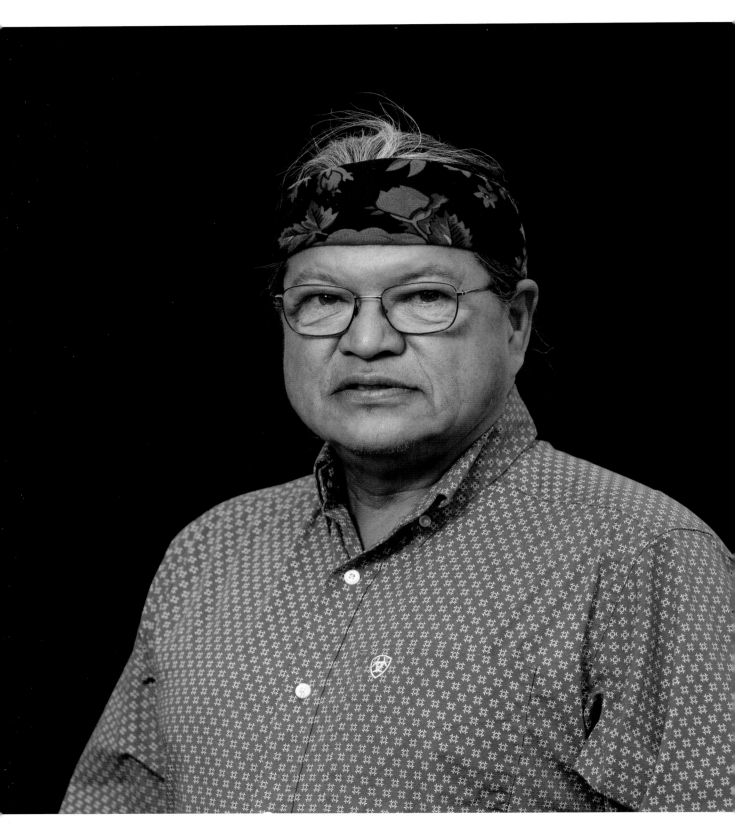

Use of Feathers to Bless Yourself and Relieve Pain

Patrick Scott
Diné (Navajo) ✳ United States

You can bless with feathers,
like the feathers we use of a bald eagle.

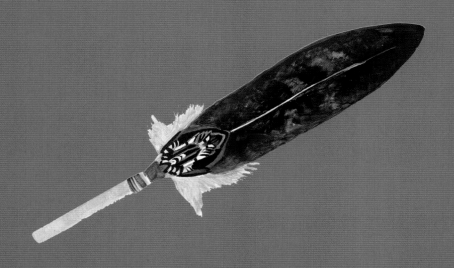

It should be noted that Indigenous Peoples undertake deep
spiritual initiations to gain the right to own bald eagle
feathers, and they can request to do so legally in the United
States. Readers are advised never to buy a feather of a bird
that has been killed, and they are encouraged to find their
feathers in nature or bird sanctuaries.

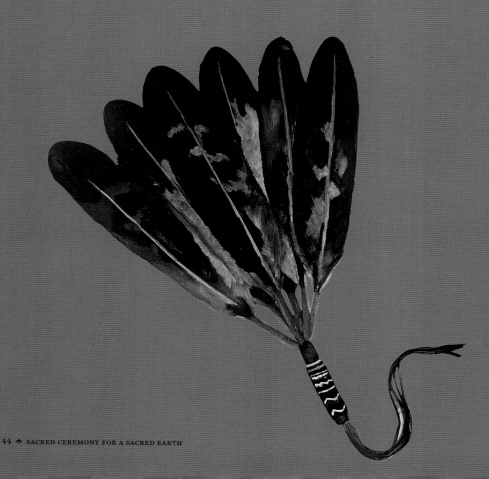

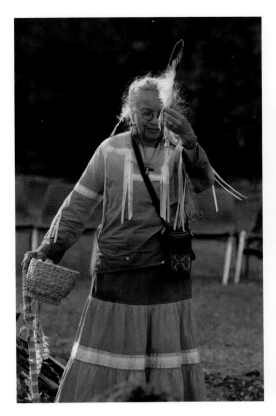
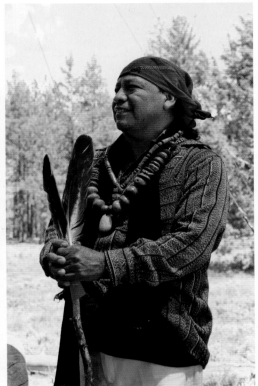

It doesn't have to be a certain type of feather—we use many different types of feathers. Different tribes have different feathers. Feather fans are a different thing. There are so many different ways to put feathers together, but the movements are really the same. You do this with a waving and bouncing motion over what you are blessing, like your altar in front of you, or over your body to bless yourself.

If you want to take something out of your body, use a sweeping motion, then send it away by blowing into the feather. Some older, traditional ways are to heat up the feather stems and point them, circle them, and sing with them, then use the sweeping or brushing motion. This is for when there's pain in your joint. For harsh problems, we would put the feather on the fireplace and hold it to and rub it around the body. These are some of the healing movements we have.

There are some ways to wave feathers toward the sky to bring clouds and the mists down to the ground. You can bring your feather to your altar or sit out in nature and hold your feather to your mouth and talk into the feather. There are deities that hear you. These are the messengers of our nation. The way Tibetans chant, we have our wisdom to talk like that too.

Hold your feather up to the sky in the morning time and shake it, then bless yourself with it.

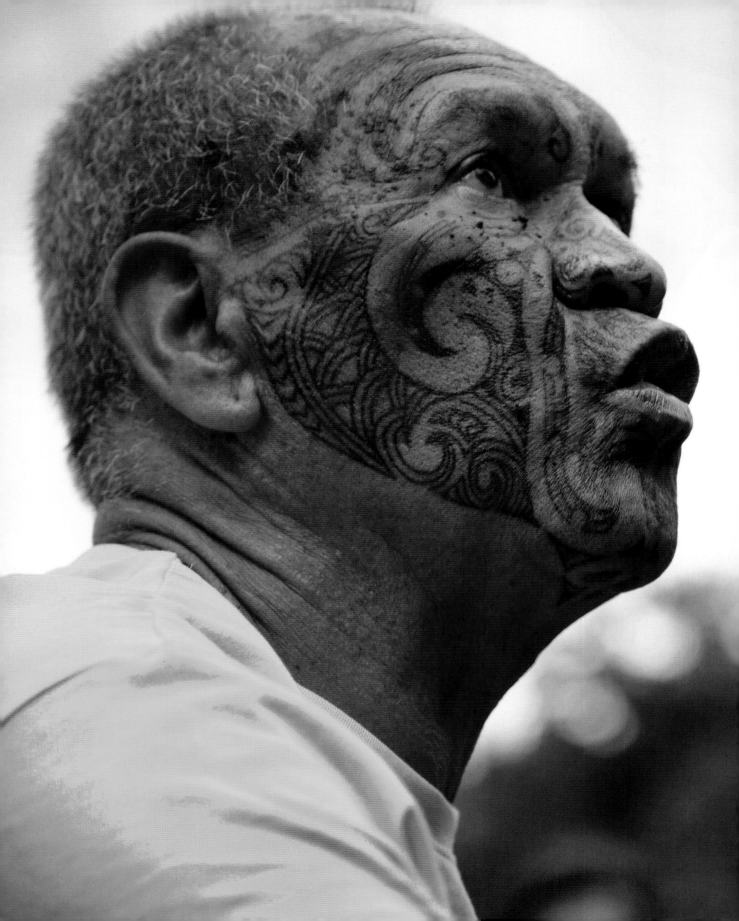

The Meaning of Sacred Face Markings

Louis Te Kouorehua Kereopa (Matua)
Māori ✳ New Zealand

The whole face represents the sky.
Everything of the heavens and everything of Earth.

The name of my "moko" (forehead markings) that I share with you is "reflection." When you look at me or when we look at each other, we see reflections of each other—not in what we see, but what we feel in our hearts. My whole face has to do with my saying yes to why I came here to Earth to be of service. Some people ask, "Can you tell me about your face?" and I'll say, "Well, if you're prepared to sit down for two hours, I'll share with you." It's so expansive.

At the bottom part of my face, my lips and what's around my mouth, there's a connection to Pachamama. Speaking. Speaking as a human, as a mortal human being on this Earth. What comes out of the mouth must not be an ego journey. Wherever I travel or whatever work I do, because this mouth speaks, it must always start from the word, which is the voice of Pachamama, our earthly voice.

My nose is the heart of the breath. That keeps me alive. It's also the heart of the spirit. On either side of my cheeks, there are patterns to do with my journey as a living spring. I don't classify myself as a master, or what they call a "shaman," or anything. No, I'm a living spring of understanding and of knowledge to the level that keeps my head above the water. The patterns are the different paths I will walk or have walked, and more to come.

On my nose, going up to my forehead, is the heart line of the connection from Pachamama to Rangi, the Sky Father of the heavens. This path, you may see it, is clear. My moko doesn't cross over it. My heart line, my connection from Pachamama to the Creator, has to be clear all the time so that when channeling comes through, when downloading comes through, the road has to be clear. It stops at the mouth so I'm able to express whatever I've been tapped on the shoulder to say. It has to be pure. It has to be clear.

That's speaking your truth—the sacred joy of truth. So, in a nutshell, that's my moko. My moko doesn't belong to me. It belongs to everyone. That's why it's called a mirror reflection, because I take joy in sitting in the presence of other people rather than them sitting with me. That's to be present. Whatever your service, to be totally present because you're that voice box. You're the voice box of the Creator. Allow that channel to be clear so that when you speak, you won't remember what you said afterward. That's being that voice. Not being aware of it, you just be you; what you do with what you do and what you have to do. You just go like the river, like the living spring. Just let it flow, because the water runs over everything and nothing can stop water.

That's my moko reflection.

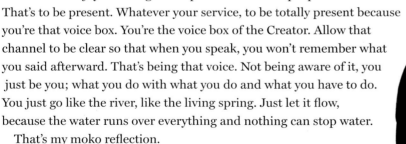

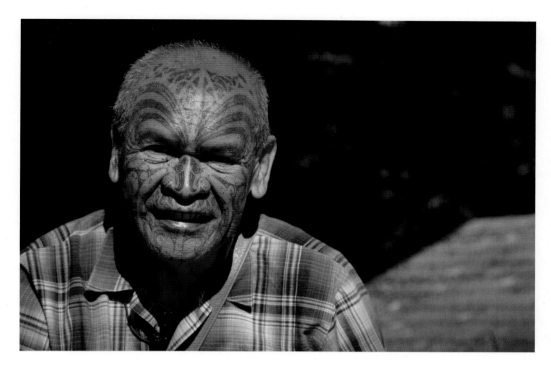

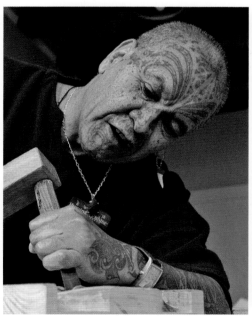

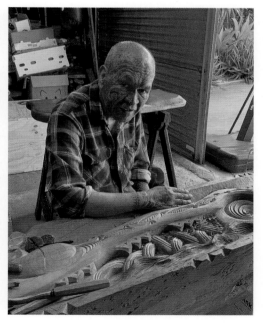

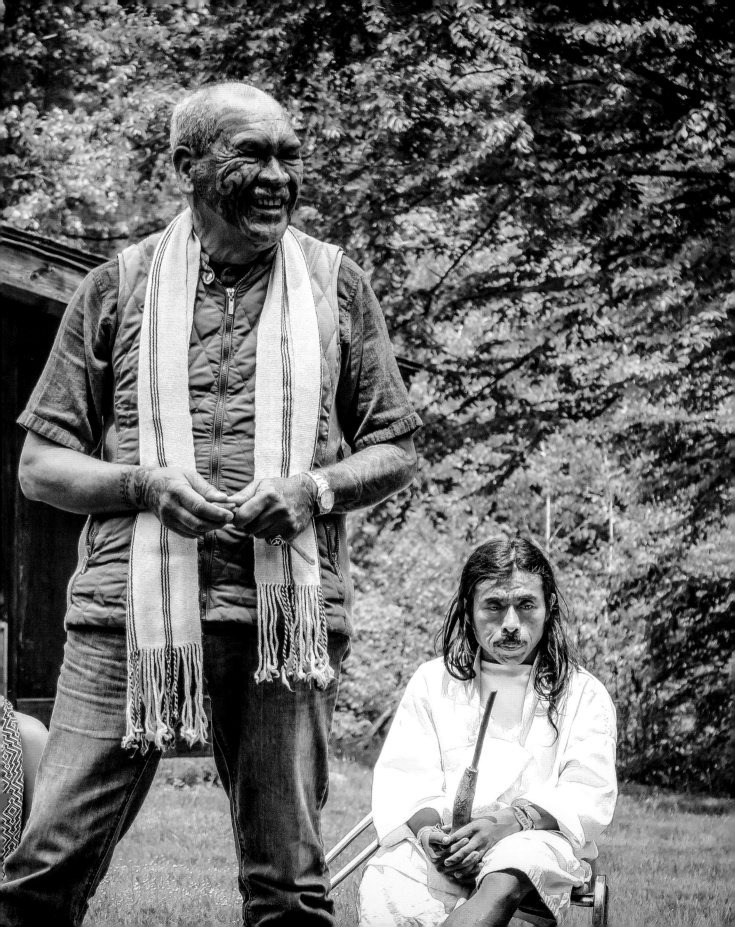

LOUIS TE KOUOREHUA KEREOPA (MATUA)

Māori ✳ New Zealand

Louis Te Kouorehua Kereopa, known as Matua, is a revered Māori elder (kaumātua) and a natural counselor and mentor, offering spiritual and emotional guidance and healing rooted in Māori wisdom and traditions. Matua teaches "Te Rakau Rangima-rie," a form of open-eyes prayer meditation honoring the Creator and Mother Earth.

Matua is also a musician and a Tohunga, or master carver, celebrated for his artistry and dedication to his craft. He was given a blessing from his elder brother to wear his facial markings, or Mono Kanohi, for his family (see page 48), representing his service of love as a Matapuna, a living spring. A close friend who is also an experienced carver executed the Ta Moko using a modern tattoo gun.

Matua's carved Māori poles, known as Pouwhenua, represent ancestral lineage, spiritual guardianship, and stories of cultural significance serving as tangible connections to the past and guides for the present and future generations.

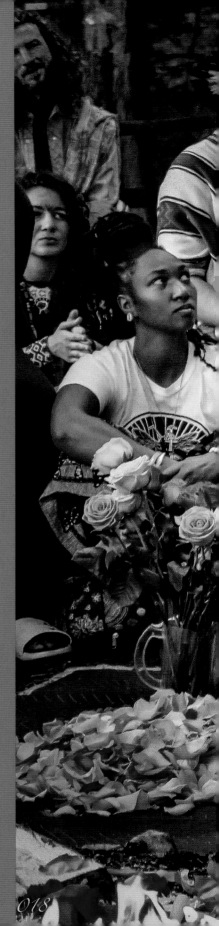

Medicine
Journeys and Messages

❋

Medicine is magic. There are energies within each of us ready to unfold, to empower our participation in all of creation. Hear from our elders about how they approach medicine as the pure essence of sacred message to be received and given through divine presence. Learn from the experiences of calls answered to find and activate the magic your medicine brings.

———•·•———

Notice what and how the elders speak about medicine through journeys and messages.

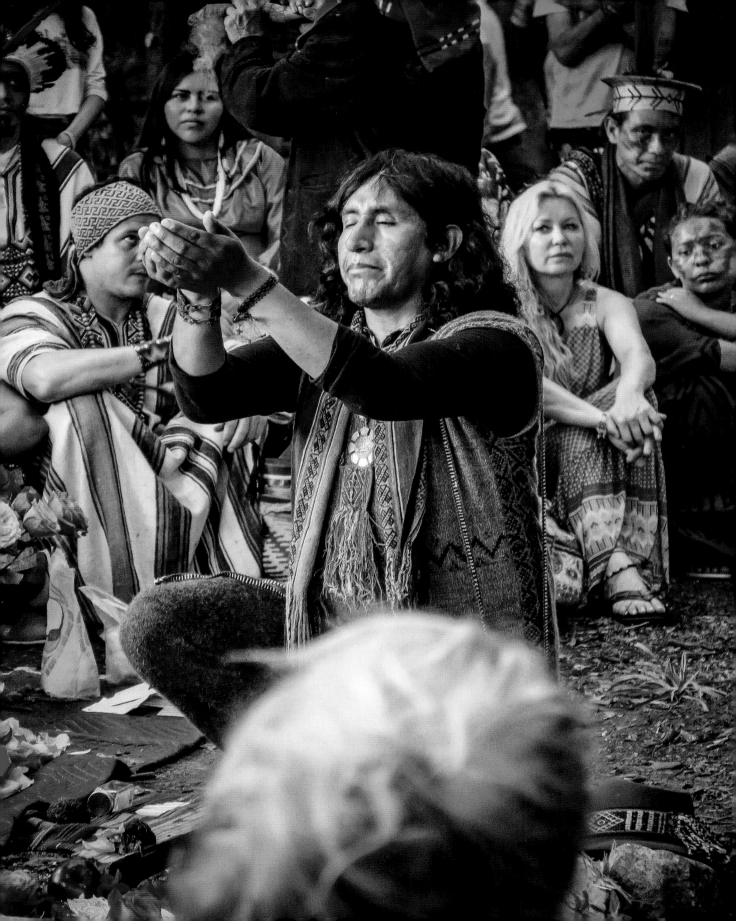

Journeying to Medicine

Túpaq Ttito Kuntur
Paq'o, Andino * Peru

Greetings from all the elders from different sites of wisdom.

A big hug from my heart.

It is a great pleasure to share with you this sacred knowledge from the land of the Inkas and Paqos ancestors. Today, I am going to share with you the wisdom of medicine, which we call "Inka Hampi." This is a secret code of Inka medicine. Medicine contains a lot of wisdom from different forms of consciousness at different levels of consciousness, coming from different worlds, known and unknown. The Inka ancestors had this ability and had the strength and wisdom to connect with the cosmic worlds in the medicine embedded in their being.

Specifically, the elders, according to their call, had a power and the gift of understanding and communicating with the cosmic beings in the Andes. Not all ancestors had the same gifts and abilities. Each had its own function in Tawantinsuyu, the four sacred regions of the Inkas that are also the four solar paths of cosmic medicine.

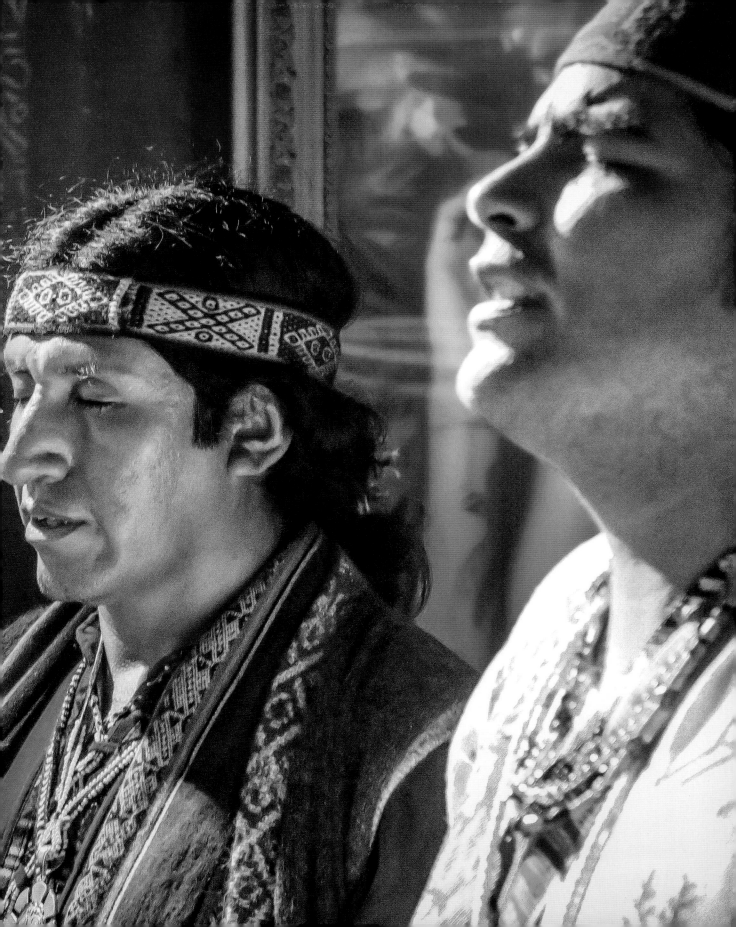

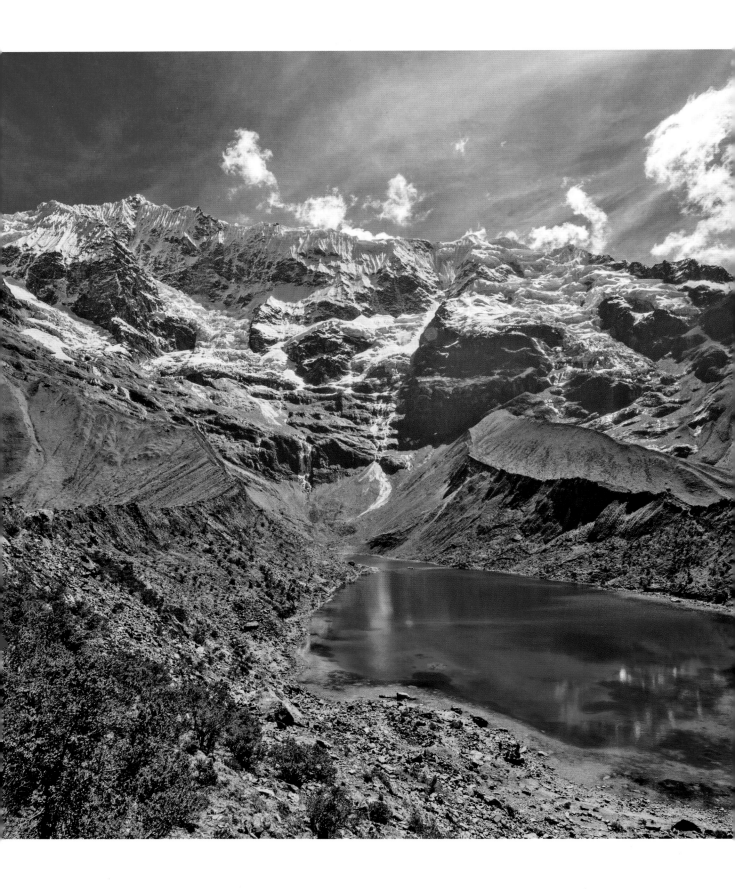

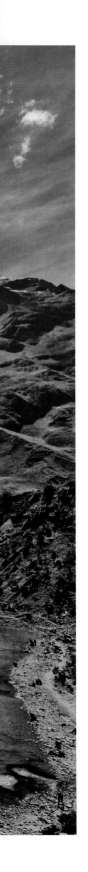

Some communicated with a bird that opened these cosmic sources of medicine to heal humanity. The elders called this bird Kuntur Hampi, which was an Apu. He would fly very discreetly through the skies here on Earth. "Hampi Apu" means "medicinal spirit" that has the sacred power of healing. Hampi Apu was not the only spirit who had this medicine. There are other spirits (Apus from the mountains and other dimensions) who have this medicine and the cosmic gift of healing. These are the spirits of medicine. Some are in this space, in this dimension, and others live beyond this dimension. Being able to reach and connect with these beings depends on our preparation in cosmic medicine. It depends on each person or each student. How can you start the path of medicine to connect and build medicine in your being?

Here in the Andes it is not easy to make the pilgrimage to connect and learn sacred medicine. I think the same thing happens with other cultures, not of the elders, but of the sacrifice to make the spiritual pilgrimage and make the physical, energetic, mental, and emotional sacrifice to cultivate and receive the gift of medicine from these beings. Here in the Andes, since the ancestors, it has always been a sacrifice to seek and connect with cosmic medicine. At this time, we continue the search for connection with cosmic medicine. We continue to learn and connect with different levels of medicine and are exploring other forms of medicinal essences. We never stop learning. We continue to learn every time we explore, every time we study, and every time we wake up, as more and more diseases also appear in people.

This teaching of medicine must be shared. We need to connect with our brothers and sisters in need around the world. We cannot keep medicine in our world and on our sacred altars. We have to interact with medicine. We have to share it. And so the medicine will continue to come from the cosmos, from the Apus.

So here in the land of the Inkas, since our ancestors, we have come and continue exploring different types of cosmic medicine. To explore and learn more, I have had to travel many times to the mountains to sacred places to have a sacred encounter. On each of my trips the experience is never the same. I always have different experiences in my being, in my consciousness, because each encounter with a sacred place of a mountain spirit is very different. In my sacred pilgrimage with medicine, I have learned that everything is medicine for me. Even a stone, no matter how simple it may seem, is medicine for me. I have discovered that the medicine is active. It's alive. It is conscious in the cosmos. There is a basic level of medicinal energy always present in nature, in the cosmos always there, contacting, touching. Much of the time we are not aware of it, so we do not connect, do not interact with this Andean medicine.

When I was a child, my grandfather told me, "Touch those plants, touch the river water, and you will be healed." And I asked, "But how is it going to heal me if it is something physical?" I didn't understand it because I was a child, but little by little, as I grew older, I understood from my grandfather that he was referring not only to physical medicine, but also to the energetic part of cosmic medicine. Following my grandfather's teachings, I began to understand beyond the physical parts of medicine and beyond the medicinal energies— that everything we touch and consume physically and energetically is medicine. We just have to know whether it has chemicals or contamination. Everything that does not have chemicals, everything that does not have pollution is good for our health, for our physical body, and for our energy.

This is a code that teaches us to understand the multidimensional essence of medicine. It is in different things that exist in the cosmos—from the simplest to the most complicated.

During this process, T'inkuy Pacha becomes fundamental since it means connection, interaction; contact with our ancestors, our cosmic beings, our sacred energies and with cosmic medicine. Today, we are in difficult times and, for many people, life becomes more difficult due to the contamination of mental and emotional consciousness and the illnesses and conflicts and other contaminations that one feels one is going through at this moment; that one is experiencing right now. Here in the Andes, we say "¡Hucha!" to all types of contamination, both physical, energetic, mental, and emotional, among others.

Many of us do not accept, do not believe, or do not want to hear these messages. There are many who are suffering right now: adults, youth, children, and the elderly. So they come to fill a void and do not remain complete, nor are they whole for themselves and for their environment. There is no spiritual or conscious discipline. Things are changing more and more. That's sad. That is worrying for our ancestors. There are young people who have woken up and understand and see this, and it is sad for them. There are prejudices and conflicts, both on personal and interpersonal levels. Since they get too carried away by stories, as well as by superficial and material things, they do not want to interact, they do not want to connect, and they do not want to have that beautiful and sacred encounter with nature, with the cosmos, or want to remember our ancestors anymore.

They feel trapped and alienated in that Hucha (negative energy) environment, in that environment of contamination; so what I want to make you aware of is something basic that can work, if you put it into practice and contact it. Given this, what method can we take to gradually get out of this mental, emotional, and physical contamination, among others? We can begin to learn or reconnect to the path of our ancestors' practices and ceremonies. Gradually practice simple steps daily or weekly or monthly, as your time allows and as you can find time to do them.

The Practice

For this practice you must find or observe a sacred place. A place where there are no distractions—maybe in your house, a space or a garden. Those who don't have that space can go to nature. Maybe when you have gone out for a walk you have seen a silent place, a sacred place. You can go to that place.

To go to that place to carry out the practice, you cannot wear street or home clothes. You have to wear some traditional ceremonial clothes or some new clothes; maybe white or a significant color. This will help reflect your energy. It will open and restart your power. Such clothing should be worn in a sacred sense, not to be taken out on the street or to the market, but to be worn when visiting sacred places or for this practice or for sacred ceremonies.

Bring flowers, sacred fruits, or seeds. What flowers do you like? Each of us has a taste for the colors of flowers. Bring a bouquet of flowers you are passionate about, that please you, that come from your heart, that inspire you, that transmit energy to you, that open you to that world of connection, to that world of ancestors, to that world you dream of and imagine. Flowers symbolize love and passion. It's part of the connection. You can work with flowers for different functions but, in this case, it is to open and reset your energy. It is the gift of your heart to cosmic beings, to ancestors or to nature.

Remember, it's connection. It's interaction. It is entering the cosmic and spiritual path.

Another point you can consider before doing the practice in the sacred place is to fast. This will help a lot in this practice. Before going out to that sacred place, you can take that day to fast. For some, only water or only natural juice. For others, they can eat some natural foods like vegetables and juices. This is cleansing your energy in your body. The cells, the neurons are waking up. They are purifiers. When we fast, we channel our energies. It does not release energies; it purifies energies. That's good. Others who already have this practice can fast for 2 or 3 days. That would be spectacular, but for those who are not used to fasting or who do not have a fasting practice, I recommend only one day a month or only the day you are visiting a sacred place. In the afternoon, when the ceremony is over, perhaps eat some natural food or some soup. May your stomach, your health, your body, your energy be well. Thus, fasting will also allow you to access the sacred space so you can do your ceremony or practice in the indicated place.

With this practice, one has to free oneself from Hucha, or negative energy, from confusion, from distractions. Do it with heart, with faith, with love. That is what our cosmic beings want. That's what our ancestors wanted. Let's open that path and portal, that sacred energetic space. We are going to connect with that cosmic energy, with that energy of nature, with the medicinal energy of plants and ancestors.

This cannot be done just once and that is enough. Do it little by little. This ceremonial practice has no limits. How do you feel this energy calling for this practice? How do you feel that call, that connection from your ancestors, from our Inka ancestors? From the cosmos? Everything depends a lot on your faith, your love, your consciousness. All this leads to the place you are going to visit. That is the point. What are we going to do there? Yes, I know you're wondering.

Being in that place, you are in a sacred space. You will see the plants, the trees, the flowers of the ancestors or the mountain or the sacred lagoon. That space is only between you and the sacred elements. Like the sacred wind. The sacred wind will listen and contact you, the spirit of water or the spirit of the plants will help you open to contact. Just between them and you. It's good to be there. You just have to be prepared with your energy centers in harmony to open up in connection. This practice is universal. I invite you to put it into practice. It is open to everyone. You just have to put it into practice.

In that sacred place it will be just you and nature. To enter that space you have to ask for permission. Therefore, you must first say your full name, where you live, and ask for permission. Three or 5 minutes are enough.

For example, you can say, "I, your daughter [say your full name], am present here and I ask your permission to access this space, your sacred space. Please receive me at this present moment, please receive my invocations, and receive a gift I brought you with a lot of love . . ."

When you arrive at the place, the energy feels different; if you feel it, go to that portal, put the flowers there, put everything that is part of the altar there—the flowers, seeds, fruits, or sacred messages you carry.

Then, sit in a comfortable place and position your body well, between the Earth and the sky, and do a meditation. In the Andes, we call "Ch'innn," which means being in the depths of silence, closing your eyes and letting the energies flow. You have to concentrate on silence and light. Silence opens. The light of Ch'innn reflects the being and the centers of it. Breathe with that reflection of Ch'innn and this will open the portals, from the inside and the outside, from inside to outside and from outside to inside. During this process, repeat about seven times, or more, "Ch'innn." Do it slowly and fluidly. This will help release the energies you have thought about, and, at the same time, you will also help release those energies that are not yours and, on the other hand, help fortify and integrate your own energies.

Alternatively, you can work with the Wajharikuy (invocation) in the sacred place, within Ch'innn or outside the Ch'innn, you can do the invocation. In the invocation, you must express, depending on how you feel, what you need for your cosmic body. Perhaps you are in poor health or perhaps you have problems; perhaps you are going through a difficult time with your partner, family, or some type of trauma. In the invocation, you can speak out loud or silently, but you have to manifest it to that sacred space and to the star of that place. You are going to communicate through that place to a cosmic being—it is like communicating with a cell phone, but it is something magical. Technology advances a lot, but our cosmic spiritual technology is more advanced. You just have to believe it. You simply have to have faith, love, and trust in what you are going to do, and communicate. This is how this summoning secret works. After finishing the invocation in that space, you can give a gift and then you can dedicate a song or play a melody, depending on how you feel in your heart for that sacred space and your soul.

This way, you can free yourself and disconnect from those Hucha, from those contaminations, from those sufferings and sadness. Perhaps three sessions, four sessions. Little by little, it is being cleansed—but it is not overnight. Everything is a process and you have to be patient. Wait, little by little, and you will feel it. This is real. Just explore and work with desire and love by opening and putting your heart, your spirit, and your energy at your disposal. Trust what you are doing because your communication and your energy are like water, like a deep ocean. When you open it, you are opening, you are moving your energy. You are receiving. Little by little, you enter and the cosmic beings, the ancestors, observe and receive you, little by little. The cosmic beings and ancestors, according to their function, will come to assist you and cleanse you, little by little.

Then, you can deliver the flowers (you can deliver the flowers before or after). You can leave them by a tree or by a rock. Don't put them in water. You can make a circle with stones. That means a lot. You are manifesting your dedication and your love with the circle of your life, your intention, your return. Don't hand it over without talking to the place. Always talk. The connection is continuous. Connection. Communication and expression.

Most people in the world have disconnected from their tradition, from their spiritual culture of the cosmos. That is why we have to return, and it is important to cleanse ourselves, purify ourselves, and free ourselves. We have to be aware of this, sisters and brothers.

Connect to medicine, connect to change.

From the Andes, I send invocations and songs on behalf of our cosmic beings and our Inka ancestors, so you have a good practice, healing, awakening, and for your connection with the sacred cosmos and your ancestors.

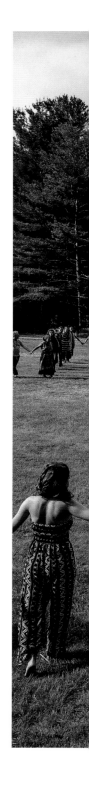

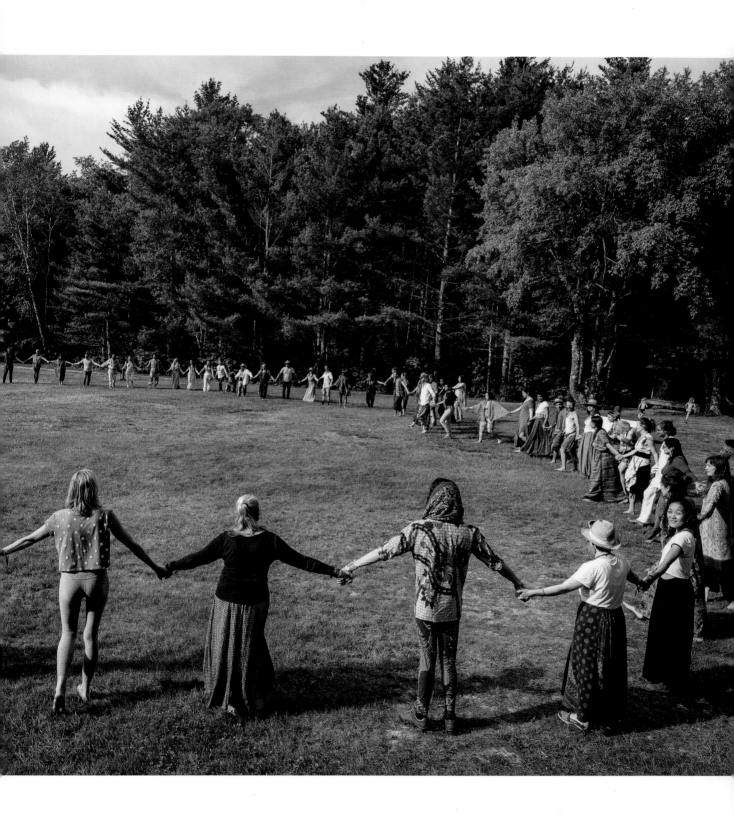

Ruawiku, Spiritual Father of Alcohol

Rodrigo Kakamukwa, as it was given to him by Mamo Jose Martin Barros
Wiwa ⁂ Sierra Nevada of Santa Marta, Colombia

This is a sacred story for the Mamos.

Sacred stories are healing. When you read a sacred story, its words are charged with energy. To do this appropriately, take two cotton balls, one in each hand, and hold them between the thumb and index finger throughout the whole story. At the end, these will be your offering to Mother Earth because they will be infused by the story's energy. By reading this story, you are doing ceremony. This is Pagamento.

All the Sierra Tribes consider alcohol as a being, as a person. There is a reason for the existence of alcohol as well as all plants and, particularly, the Teacher Plants: marijuana, ayahuasca, etc. All the sacred plants are there for a reason. It's important for us to know how to interact with them. Sometimes, if we don't know how, it will create problems for us, particularly mental problems. Our interaction with alcohol and the Teacher Plants will affect the mind.

One of many ways to do Pagamento, or a ceremony for alcohol, is by invoking or listening to the sacred story of Ruawiku, the Spiritual Father of Alcohol.

Ruawiku was one of the Spiritual Fathers in nature who had many wives. He was married to trees and plant species that carry the feminine energy, such as different types of fruit trees. All the trees that bear sweet fruit are feminine trees. Ruawiku was also married to all the cane and vine species in nature, such as sugarcane and ayahuasca.

He was a very powerful Spiritual Father who performed miracles.

Ruawiku was not only a Spiritual Father in nature, but also the Spiritual Father of all the Little Brothers, the Westerners. He had several children, sons and daughters. Each child was born out of his pain and sacrifice. He has the authority to act on behalf of the Creator of all the tribes of the Sierra. And, in this capacity, he had healing abilities and could intercede on people's behalf before the Creator. Ruawiku would order and implement all the principles the Creator had given, putting them into practice. Because of that, many people did not like

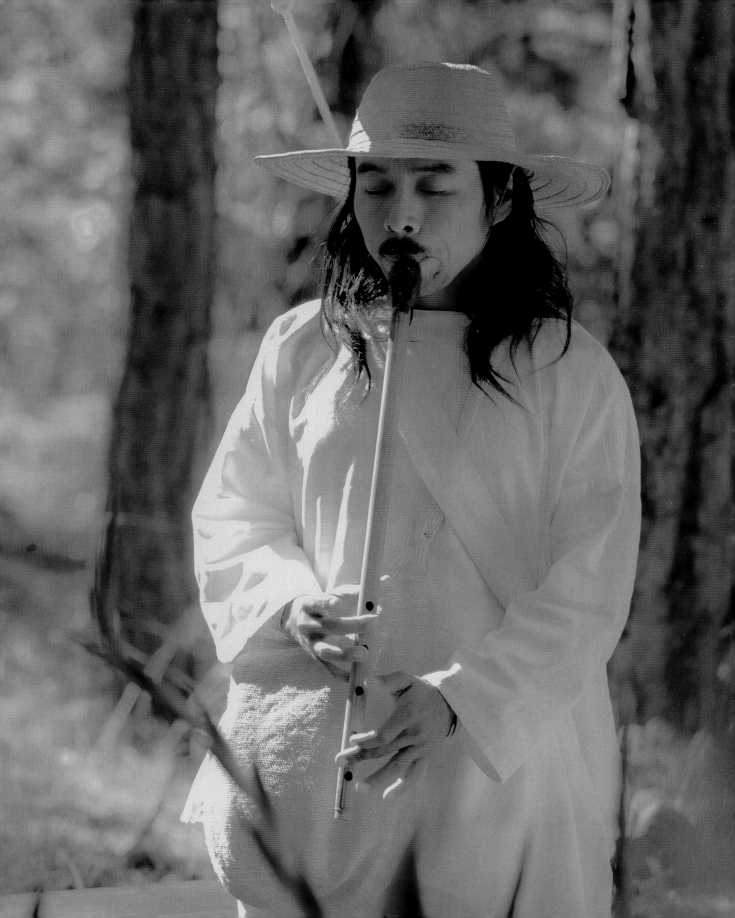

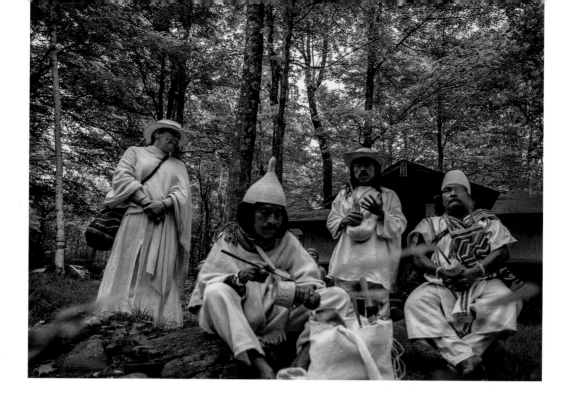

Ruawiku. He faced a great deal of opposition and pain inflicted on him by the people in positions of power. He was a rebel who wanted to help and heal the people who needed it.

Ruawiku was under constant persecution by those in power who disagreed with his beliefs. The final intent of this endless persecution was to kill Ruawiku. He was very powerful and, as a result, had many enemies who used to team up against him. Every time he was hit by his enemies, and, with every punch he received, shedding tears and spilling blood, miracles were born out of his blood and tears. Out of these drops, new species of plants were born, a new daughter was born with each drop.

Ruawiku daughters were called Nengulas, and they were very different in appearance. Among his daughters, there were red-haired, blonde, and brunette Nengulas with different complexions and features. However, they were very similar in nature—they all were independent, rebellious, and extremely wise. They also were powerful healers and could heal different types of problems people may have. With each daughter born, a different type of vine, or cane, or fruit tree was created.

When someone is drinking alcohol, the person is, without knowing, interacting spiritually with Ruawiku and is also spiritually seeking a sexual encounter with one of Ruawiku's daughters. That explains why it is important to ask for forgiveness from Ruawiku or permission to court one of his daughters, and this can be done by doing Pagamento, a ceremony, for alcohol.

Ruawiku is the doctor who brings to us all types of medicine.

Ruawiku, as a powerful Spiritual Father, will help you control the effects and cravings of alcohol. A Pagamento, or a ceremony for alcohol, helps people who have anger issues, people with addictive personalities, people who speak impulsively or without thinking (like intoxicated people often do). It will also have a beneficial effect in nature, particularly for plant species such as canes, vines, and fruit trees. By reading or listening to this sacred story, you are honoring Ruawiku, the Spiritual Father of Alcohol. This sacred story is better to be shared when in nature under a fruit tree, and, when doing so, call upon the presence of the spirits of Ruawiku as well as the Spiritual Father Mukueke, who used to work in partnership with Ruawiku.

There are two main characters in this story: one is logical, representing the positive principles of the creator, such as order; the other (who is not named) represents anarchy, jealousy. This principle was what created the sugarcane. From that sugarcane, we make alcohol. There are two principles in the world, but we don't judge them. They exist. The sugarcane we make alcohol from carries the negative principle. It was not meant to be drunk regularly. It is the same with alcohol made from fruits. They are only created to be consumed to do Pagamento, or ceremony. It is like a prescription from a doctor to clean the negativity from us by drinking with measure and care and authorization.

Young people are not given authorization to consume alcohol or any other sacred plants. It's not because of the physical damage alcohol or marijuana or other sacred plants could have on the physical body—that's not the main reason. The main reason is that they uncover a type of knowledge. It's not good for the soul. Every time we drink, we need to know the reason we are drinking. When we drink, we gather materials. We take these things and carry them within us, which makes our souls heavy. When you take things from a store, you pay for them at the register. This is exactly the same. We cannot take any of these spiritual materials without doing Pagamento ceremony to the Spiritual Father. If we don't do that, we are generating a debt. It becomes cumulative and it gets worse gradually.

If you keep drinking without measure, you are going to say things or do things that are very negative. People create problems or get into trouble because they are under the effects of whatever substance they're using. Our souls get heavy because we carry the energy of this negativity with us in our field, and it is contagious. If your soul is heavy, if your soul is carrying negative things, even if you have not drunk that day, you are transmitting it into the environment with other people.

Carrying these energies with us reflects something very important: the Nine Levels of Human Thought. This ancestral knowledge relates to the nine planets and the nine layers of Earth. They are interconnected with the Nine Levels of Human Thought. We will share only three: anger, lies, and anxiety.

When we talk with anger, we are damaging the truth. We are damaging good people just by using words when we are angry. The anger is not in someone else. The anger, in reality, is within each of us and that's the reason we react. If we don't have anger within us, if we have cleared the anger in our field, people could say anything to us and we won't react.

Anger is like fire. Our planet has fire inside. If we let the fire out, it damages not only the people we express our anger toward, but also the Earth. We are creating an imbalance. If we all are angry and we all are speaking angry words, what is going to happen with the planet? Mother Earth will show this fire as volcanic activity or heat waves. Anger equals fire. If the whole human race is angry, it will have an effect on the weather; it will have an effect on the planet. We need purification for this imbalance. We need to go through a process to balance these layers of thoughts through words, music, and Pagamento ceremony.

Now, take those two little pieces of cotton you are holding between your fingers and bury them at the foot of a tree (especially fruit trees or grapevines), immediately after you finish reading the story. Then, perform two full body rotations counterclockwise and leave the place.

This is Pagamento.

Pagamento for Ruawiku, Spiritual Father of Alcohol

Rodrigo Kakamukwa, as it was given to him by Mamo Jose Martin Barros
Wiwa ☀ Sierra Nevada of Santa Marta, Colombia

When we do Pagamento, or a ceremony to honor Ruawiku, the Spiritual Father of Alcohol, we a honor all the species in nature used to make alcohol, such as apples, cherries, grapes, pears, sugarcane, etc.

For centuries, we have used them without acknowledging or honoring those plant species for the wine they make, the rum they make, etc., which created an unbalanced relationship between humans and nature. As a result, we ended up owing Mother Nature, in other words we have been in debt with nature for centuries.

At a personal level, a Pagamento for Ruawiku will help break addictive behaviors such as drinking excessively or excessive use of plant medicine, and, in nature, will honor and nourish all the plant species of which Ruawiku is the Spiritual Father, such as fruit trees, all types of cane (sugarcane) and vines (ayahuasca).

A Pagamento for Ruawiku is done outdoors, ideally, but not necessarily, under a fruit tree or grapevine. You will need two little pieces of cotton that you have dipped in clear, meaning colorless, alcohol made from sugarcane, such as rum or cachaça. We will call upon the presence of Ruawiku as well as the Spiritual Father Mukueke who used to work in partnership with Ruawiku.

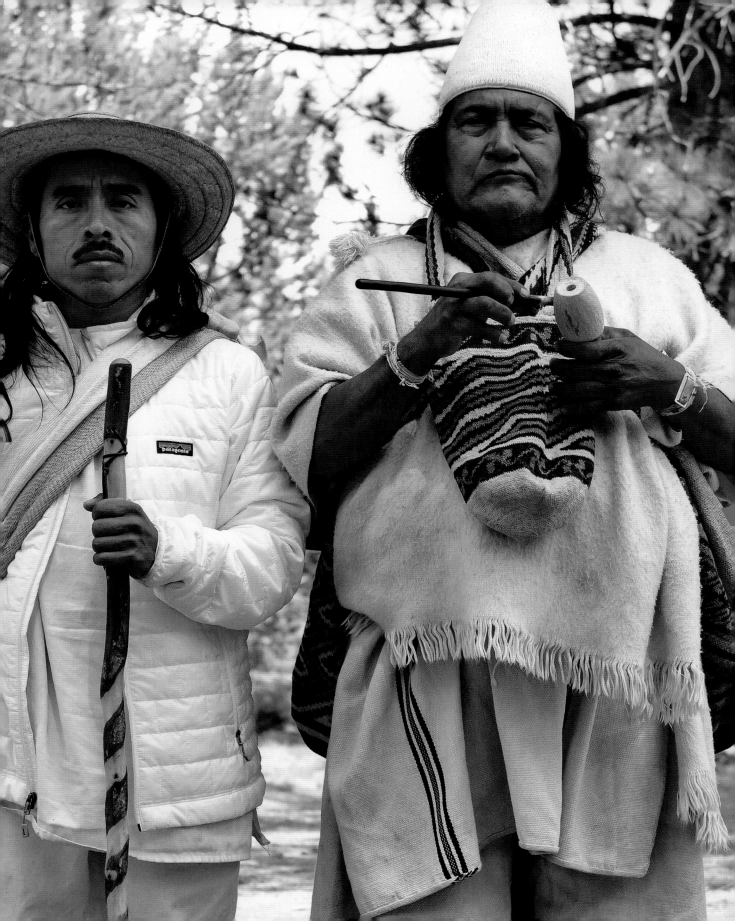

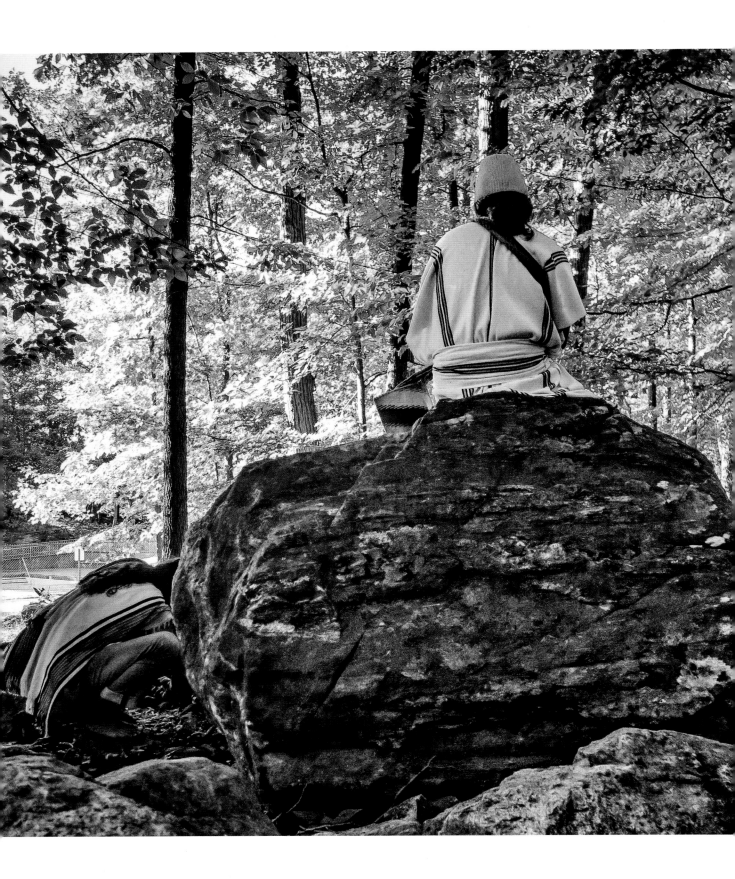

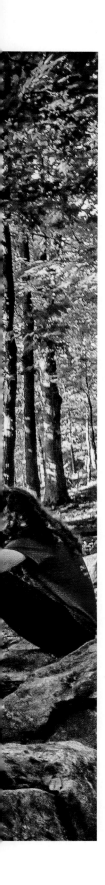

Remember, Ruawiku is the doctor who brings us all types of medicines and healing.

A Pagamento for Ruawiku involves acknowledging the duality—therefore, it requires honoring both the negative energy as well as the positive.

We live in a world of duality: day and night, man and woman. One cannot survive without the other. These opposites must be in harmony to maintain balance.

We, the Teyuna People, not only acknowledge the dual nature of our world, but also respect it.

We will first do the negative energy Pagamento.

Pagamento for the Negative

Begin by holding one of the two pieces of cotton dipped in clear alcohol (set the other aside for later use) between your index finger and thumb of the **left hand**. While holding the cotton, close your eyes for the visualization to begin.

We are going to visualize all different kinds of foods that are rotten or spoiled: Visualize rotten apples and bananas, rotten eggs, spoiled meat and fish, rancid milk and juices. After we have gathered large amounts of spoiled foods in our mind, we will visualize dollar bills that are old, crushed, and torn. We will hold these images in our mind for 10 to 15 minutes to allow the piece of cotton we are holding to become infused with the energy of rotten food and old, torn dollar bills. We will set aside this little piece of cotton infused with negative energy, then we will get the other little piece of cotton to do the Pagamento for the positive.

Pagamento for the Positive

Begin by holding the second piece of cotton dipped in alcohol between your index finger and thumb of your **right hand**. While holding the cotton, close your eyes for the visualization to begin.

We are going to visualize the finest wines we know, the most expensive brandy, Champagne, Scotch, etc. Visualize large amounts.

Imagine all types of sweet fruits—apples, cherries, grapes, pears, plums, etc.—the most beautiful fruits you can possibly imagine without blemish. Visualize large amounts.

Now, we will bring back memories of the sweet smell of perfume, as when we got close to a person who smelled wonderful. We will imagine the most beautiful clothes—high-quality blouses, coats, dresses, jackets, pants, and shoes made of luxurious fabrics. Visualize all of those expensive clothes made of gold.

We will also visualize newly minted money—bills in perfect condition, clean and with the smell of fresh, new money. Visualize large amounts.

We will hold these images in our mind for 10 to 15 minutes to allow the cotton we are holding to become infused with the positive energy of what we are visualizing.

Ruawiku needs both the positive and negative energies.

Now, gather the two pieces of cotton infused with negative and positive energies. Dig a hole at the foot of a fruit tree and bury the cotton pieces in it. Cover the cotton with soil and place a small rock on top.

Perform two full body rotations counterclockwise and leave the place immediately without looking back.

This is Pagamento.

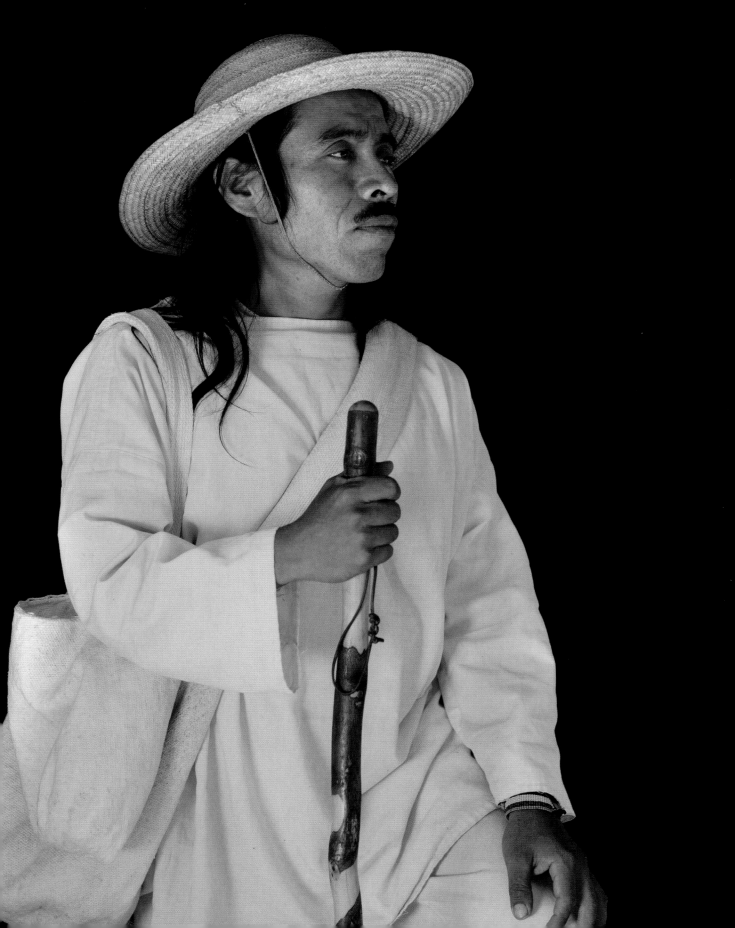

RODRIGO, SEWIGU KAKAMUKWA

Wiwa ⁂ Sierra Nevada, Colombia

Mamo Sewigu Kakamukwa (Mamo Rodrigo) comes from a lineage of Mamos that goes beyond his great-great-grandfather. His family comes from the Kakamukwa lineage and there have been Mamos in his family in every single generation.

Mamo Sewigu (Mamo Rodrigo) was an educator and leader of his community before receiving his Segwa (power object, spiritual gifts) at the head of the Jerez River when being ordained as a Mamo.

Mamo Sewigu is not only a Mamo, but he was a Maestro first.

For the Teyuna, a Maestro is a weaver, a storyteller, a musician, a teacher, and in charge of making sacred objects for the community.

A Maestro is the weaver who makes the walls of the temple and the hats the Wiwa People wear. A Maestro also makes the carrumbo (sacred object: a spindle) that the young females use to spin cotton.

Mamo Sewigu (Rodrigo) was the teacher who opened the first bilingual school in 2007 inside the Reservation to teach basic Spanish and math, as well as their traditional knowledge, to prevent the youngsters from leaving the Reservation while preserving their cultural identity. He has also worked for the Colombian Public Health Department during public health campaigns as a nurse. His knowledge of the Teyuna languages as well as his knowledge of the Wiwa and Kogi territories in the state of Guajira enables him to act in the capacity of an intercultural bridge.

Mamos are the spiritual leaders, or priests, for the Teyuna People. They are the counselors for their communities, and they perform all the important ceremonies for their people, such as weddings, funeral rites, rites of passage, and baptisms. They are also the healers and the teachers of their communities. The word "Mamo" means "enlightenment of both good and evil." Mamos hold the spiritual knowledge of their people and are trained from an early age to do healings, Pagamentos, or ceremonies, as well as divination. The word "Mamo" also means "the sun," as the sun of our solar system has the ability to illuminate all beings.

Earth
Plants and Stones

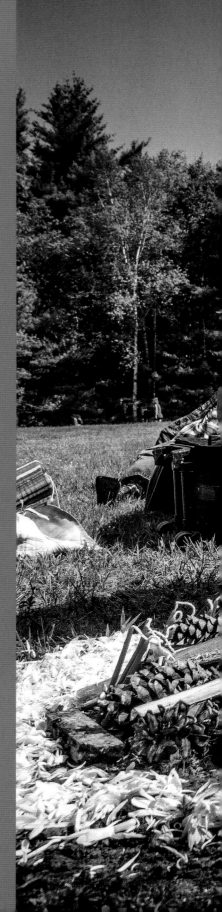

❋

Earth is the ground we walk upon, live upon, feed upon. It is nourishment at its most sacred and yet mundane. Hear from our elders about how they relate to the blessings of the soil, food, and treasures that complete our understanding of the gifts the Earth can bring.

Notice what and how the elders speak about Earth through plants and stones.

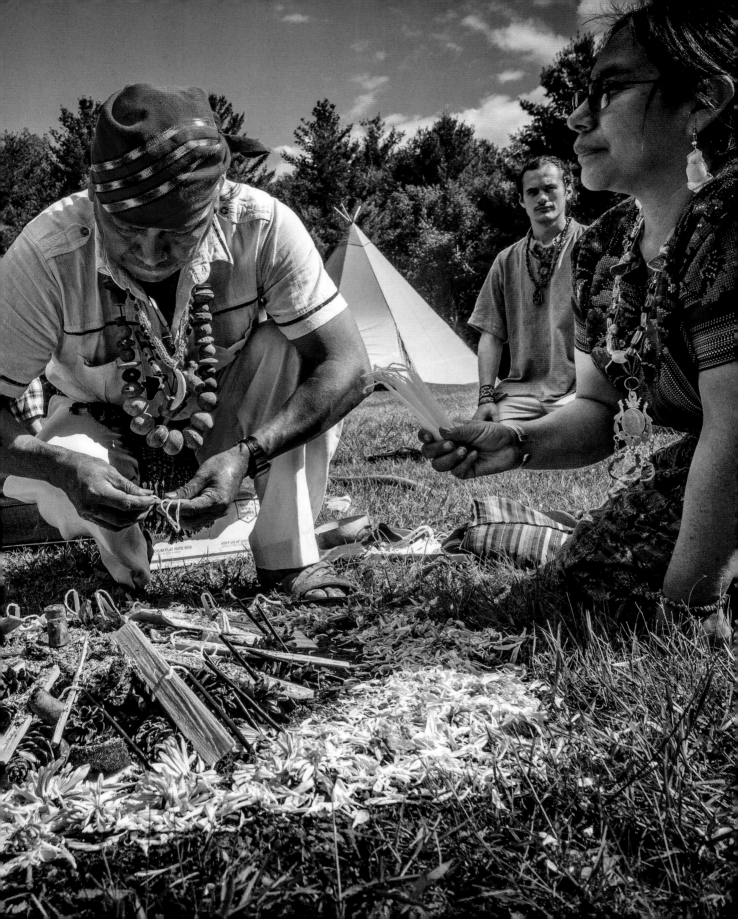

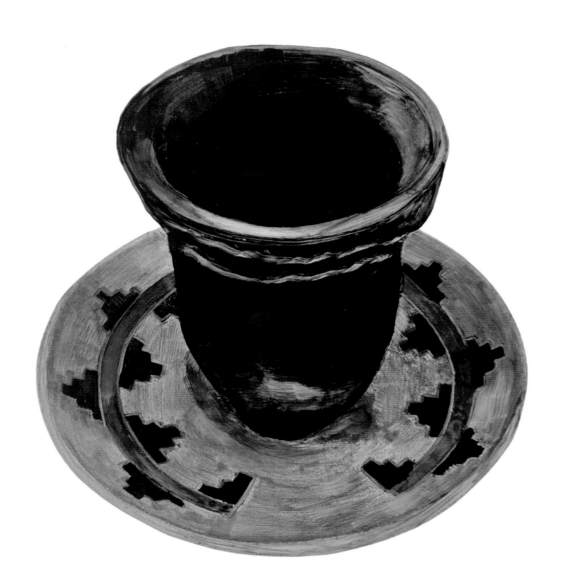

Earth and Sun Connection for Nourishing Your Body

Patrick Scott
Diné (Navajo) ✳ United States

Everything we do is on this Earth.

Mud. It's just around here where I live. The mud is really the Earth and the water, mixed up. The Earth, the universe, the waters, the mountain ranges, the forest, they're all integrated into this. It has all the different nutrients and minerals Earth offers. It has everything in there and everything that's connected. Another way of being connected with Earth is when we drink out of clay pots, it replenishes us. The medicines are one traditional method we have: we make tea into powder and then re-cook and add water and drink it. That's one of the major connections to Earth. That's the same thing as putting sand on yourself after a sweat (see page 23).

Among these Indigenous People, all the way from Alaska to Chile, it's the same. It's the same for all of us in how we use these sacred elements. These are the ways we keep connected to Mother Earth. This is the connection. Then, we sing.

Balancing Energies with Cacao

Nana Rosalía Zavala and Ixquik Zavala
Maya K'iche ❊ Guatemala

The energy of cacao connects to life.

It is from Mother Earth. Growing fruit always connects to the Earth.

When we take cacao, we have more presence with ourselves—with our purpose. That is why it always has a duality. True duality is always sought to be in balance. There is importance in knowing how to have presence in every step, in every action, in every moment. Find that inner strength. Find that inner medicine. This is why we use cacao.

We present the cacao with a candle. We always connect it to the heart. There is heat from our hearts. We say to the fire: *We are here and we are now*. Then, to the forehead:*We are here and we are now*. To the heart: *We are here and we are now*. To Mother Earth: *We are here and we are now*. Then, to the breath. Inhale. Exhale. Breathing with connection, inhaling and exhaling three times. Then, open the vocal cords. Make the connection with the ancestors. Honor the past. *Aaaaaahhhhhh.*

We always have this connection with cacao in mind, because it is in our cosmology.

It is given to the women. When you give birth, you connect with this energy of cacao.

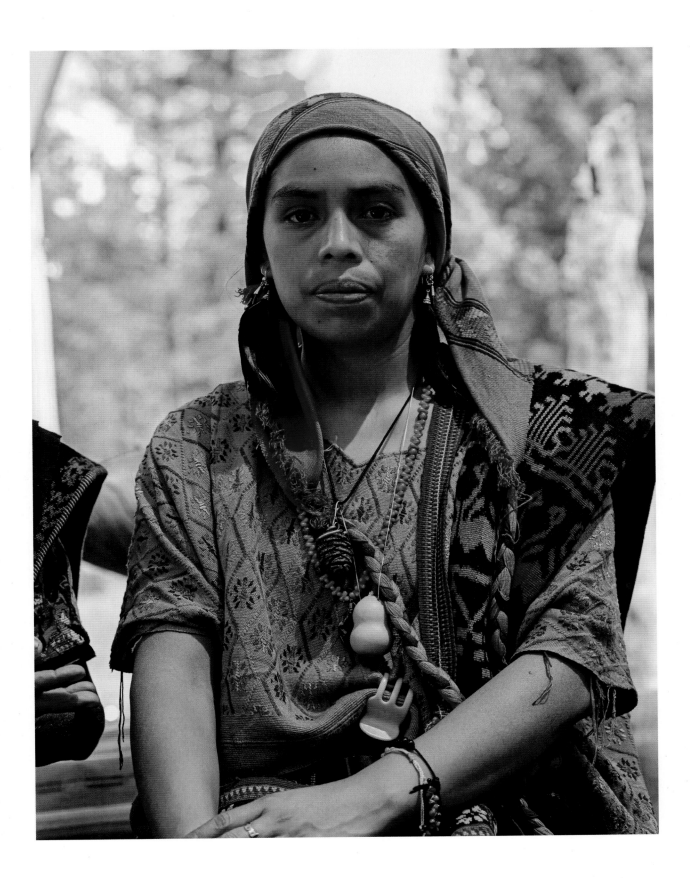

In spirituality there are various forms of offering sacred drinks to divinity. Native Peoples find the connection in the seeds the Earth produces, to be able to unify and create duality of energies that allows the balance between human life and spiritual life to achieve harmony and good living in this existence. We mix different elements with the cacao to attain that sacred duality.

- Cacao and corn
- Cacao and fermented cane juice
- Cacao and fermented fruits
- Cacao and pataxte
- Cacao and sapote seed
- Cacao and vanilla

When cacao is in the Earth, it embodies masculine energy. When it is mixed with other elements, it transforms into feminine energy, except in the case of pataxte, which embodies feminine energy. In that scenario, cacao retains its masculine energy.

For us, the cacao drink is the balance of the body, in that way the person finds the connection of heaven and Mother Earth. Per cup of hot water, we use 30 to 40 grams of 60 percent cacao powder for Earth power and 40 percent masa (ground corn) for feminine power. You can find your own balance by adding more of either ingredient as you boil it.

Duality is a balance. When we talk about cacao, the main thing for us is to understand the balance of duality. Masculine and feminine energy. Day and night. What is close, what is far away. What our eyes see and what we cannot see. Cacao brings a balance for our ancestors. It helps us detach from ourselves and from habits that don't serve us. There are so many vices. Cacao helps us leave this world that we live in a little bit. We get very involved in all that is fast, all that is disposable, but in the world of cacao medicine, we become aware and understand that we must learn to dance with life and follow the rhythm of nature. Just as flowers know their time to bloom and bear fruit, just as animals know when they need to procreate, the human being seeks that balance in their life. This is what cacao wants to tell us.

The industrial forms of cacao interrupt the spiritual connection we can have with it. There is no awareness. There are machines that take 10 to 15 minutes to do what human work and the force of the Earth take time to produce. This no longer has the same connection. This no longer has the same energy. More fertilizer and more insecticides get used according to the studies they carry out. It produces more, but it is exploited more. We relate the cacao plant to the human body of women. When there is no care, there is exploitation. This is a situation that produces pain. When we receive the medicine of cacao like this, there is no longer consciousness. From even this, the cacao teaches us how to be more aware of what is happening. Both our bodies and the body of Mother Earth are one. We have to take care of her.

Our life is only a minute in this great immense time of humanity. That's why cacao is so profound for us to understand spirituality, because as those who grow it learn, we have to be in harmony with the animals, with the butterflies, with the insects. We have to be in harmony with the worms. We have to find a way to have that balance so we can receive well and continue dancing with life. Our ancestors take us to this world of consciousness we are a part of.

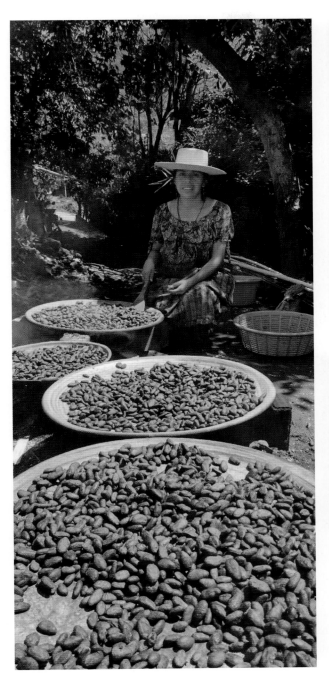
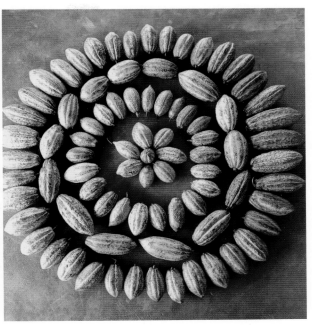
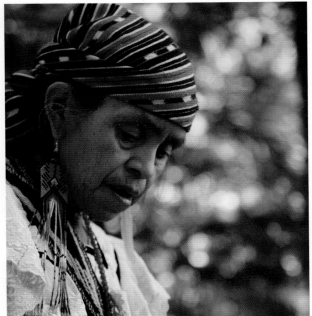

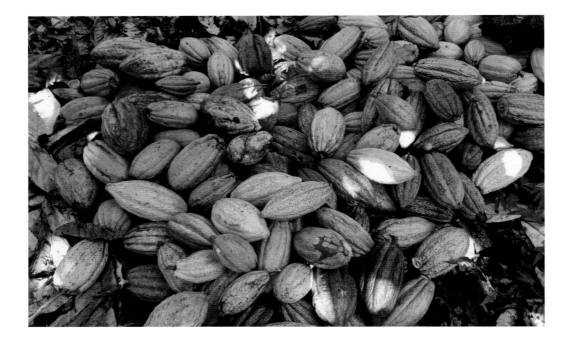

Cacao connects the energy of the Earth and is already looking for the duality that connects the energy of the universe. In that way, we understand we are all part of this ancestral medicine, and we just have to be aware. When there is awareness, there will be no abuse of medicine. We understand that our medicine is made for everyone, but we also understand what the purpose is. If we don't understand, then difficult situations come in life because we confuse ourselves and we confuse others.

In the end, our ancestors taught us something from the beginning. From our Maya worldview, it begins with the spiritual part of cacao, the seed. The principle is to connect with the spirit of each element.

In the political organization of communities, cacao is very special because it seeks to balance situations. There are conflicts in communities and in societies. Cacao is the element that shows, like the presence of serenity, an awareness that, with communication, everything can lead to harmony in the end. It takes us there.

This is our worldview. This is K'iche. This is our culture. It has always carried a history of where my grandmothers and grandfathers have been, people who have grown their cacao plant. My grandfather was a farmer who dedicated himself to astronomical study, to know when to plant and how to plant. He never used insecticides or fertilizers enough to harm the Earth, life, and whoever receives it. They always had their own way of being in harmony with the animals. The animals look for cacao to feed themselves, and we plant cacao to feed and nourish our family. This awareness asks, "What can I do to take care of life and nature?"

My grandmother was the one who prepared the cacao. She was the one who worked it on the grinding stone. That takes us to the spirit of cacao that has to do with the energy that we give it to move the forces of the Earth. Grandmothers hold that teaching, where their breasts and the release of energy from their womb connect to the Earth. That is why the grinding stone has three foundations. When the woman grabs it, she works it with a force of conscious giving and receiving.

Already knowing this process, the people, when they have conflicts, like planting or land conflict situations, they use cacao as a part of solving them. Everyone has their own way of taking care of cacao, the seed.

There are practices we still carry out, such as marriages where the reading of the cacao is done to find out if the marriage will be functional. The man is the one who brings the cacao and puts it to the test of truth with his fiancée. Then, the woman has to do the toasting over firewood and she has to peel and grind the cacao over the three stones and place it in a gourd. Once she has it in a paste, she washes her hands and uses them to beat the cacao paste, extracting oils that form shapes on its surface. Based on these shapes, a reading is conducted; we evaluate what the cacao says. The two mothers of both families are the ones to do that reading and make the evaluation. They determine if the marriage will be functional, or not. If it is functional, then the cacao that was prepared is shared with the entire family. According to what came out, they observe whether the stars, animals, plants, or some other energy that manifests in cacao determines that the relationship is not functional. Then the cacao that was prepared by the woman is returned to the family and they are told there is no marriage. These practices are still done today, but it is a decision to make. If you want to search for your life's complement, then accept the final answer.

With these cacao analyses, we get to the point in a spiritual way. There is a long training to become a spiritual guide. We have twenty energies, like twenty specialties; we talk about it in the Cholq'ij Maya calendar. It is a study, a profound science, for each energy. In this case, what is intended to be connected with is spirituality. Through our training we learn to understand the energy because we are energy and we create energy with medicine. In the end, we understand that cacao helps us harmonize our lives.

To hold a cacao ceremony for others requires training and preparation. Our ancestors always had cacao in ceremonies and in marriages with gratitude. They did this with gratitude because we are here to learn. We are grateful for the seeds they already put into the Earth. We have cacao for a birth. We have cacao for a pregnancy too. Even when someone transcends, when they die, cacao is present because we are grateful for that life that is already gone. Cacao is also used in major events, such as being grateful that the rain is coming down and returning. We have cacao when there is a lot of thunder and ask for balance. You drink cacao when you need space to work or to purify. Cacao helps us harmonize our lives.

For us, to understand the spirituality of cacao, you have to learn the language of cacao—its way of being. To understand it, you need a personal awareness. Understand that everything has a beginning and everything has an end.

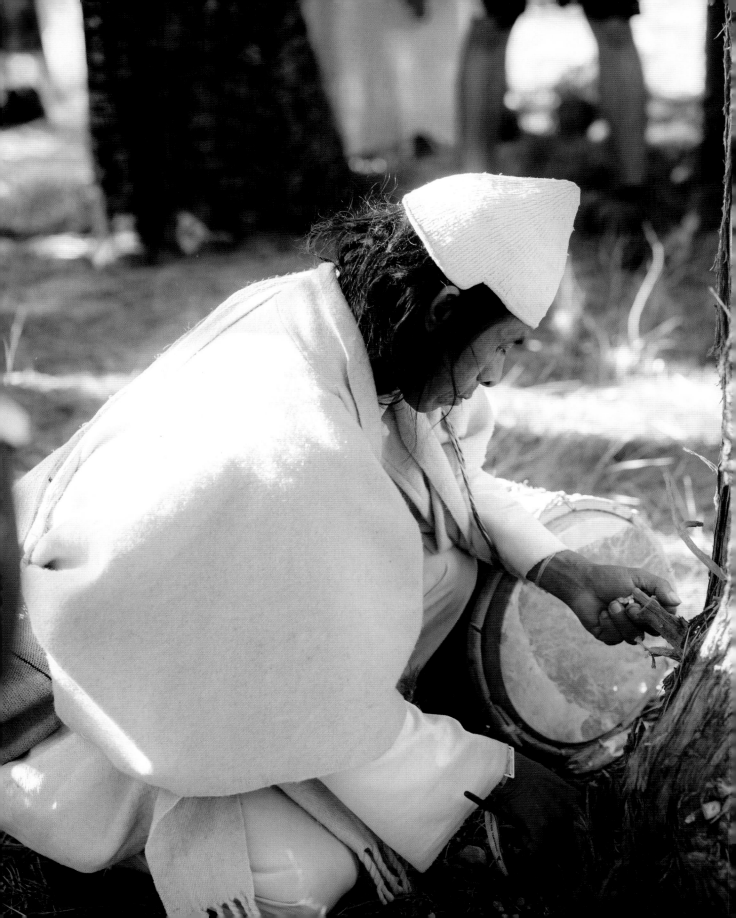

Pagamento for Trees

Rodrigo Kakamukwa, as it was given to him by Mamo Jose Martin Barros
Mamo Wiwa ✳ Sierra Nevada of Santa Marta, Colombia

Doing Pagamento in nature for trees reminds us we are connected to the trees, that we belong to nature, and we do not exist outside of nature—we are just part of nature.

It helps us connect more deeply and become more aware of nature and, consequently, kinder to the planet. Whenever we do any type of Pagamento, we also receive personal healing. During times of uncertainty, as are the times in which we live now, trees can help us in many ways.

- Trees can help us restore our ancestral memories. They can help ground us when we need it most (as when we're having an emotional overload, when going through a solar flare, a cosmic event, or when we have been over exposed to electromagnetic frequencies like Wi-Fi, cell phones, etc.).

- Trees can protect us from damaging radiation and electromagnetic pollution. Trees are affected by the Earth's magnetic field—the last collapse of Earth's magnetic field was recorded in the trunk of a 42,000-year-old kauri tree in New Zealand.

- Trees and humans have an interdependent relationship. As humans breathe in oxygen and exhale carbon dioxide, trees take in carbon dioxide and release oxygen.

- Trees have given themselves freely for the benefit of humanity since the beginning of this world. If all trees disappear from the Earth, we will die as well—we couldn't breathe the air we breathe.

When we (humans) separate ourselves from the tapestry of life thinking we are more valuable than a tree or a rock, a wild animal, we contribute to the demise of our planet and humanity.

Pagamento

Take a couple of deep breaths and pull your energy in until you feel you are in a state of both relaxation and focus.

Begin by saying "thank you" to the Spiritual Father of the trees and plants.

If you are in a forest or close to a grove, look for the oldest tree in the group. Facing this tree, go inward and ask silently for permission to be in the forest. Begin by saying, "Thank you, Kalashe, Spiritual Father of the trees and plants. I'm here before you today to give you the spiritual gifts you need."

Using your visualization skills, imagine you have the kind of "tumas" the Mamos call "Kunkwakuichi" as offerings during ceremony, or Pagamento. "Tumas" are pieces of quartz and other crystals left by the ancestors to be used by the Kogis, Arhuacos, Wiwas, and Kankuamos—the Indigenous People of the Sierra Nevada.

Besides the tumas, also visualize firewood, food, and real money, such as bills of any currency.

After a couple of minutes of focusing on the objects you will use as offerings, call upon the presence of Jose Maria Kakamukua by calling his name three times:

- ✖ Jose Maria Kakamukua,

- ✖ Jose Maria Kakamukua,

- ✖ Jose Maria Kakamukua.

Give him your visualizations as offerings, which are "tumas": food, firewood, and money.

The reason you are giving the offering to him is because he has the role of an ambassador—he acts as a bridge between Westerners and the kingdoms of nature. Jose Maria Kakamukua was a legendary Mamo of great power.

Ask Jose Maria Kakamukua to give your offering to the Spiritual Father of the plant kingdom, Kalashe.

After thanking Jose Maria Kakamukua, perform two full rotations counterclockwise with your body.

This is Pagamento.

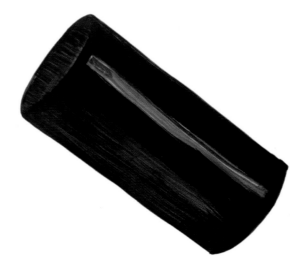

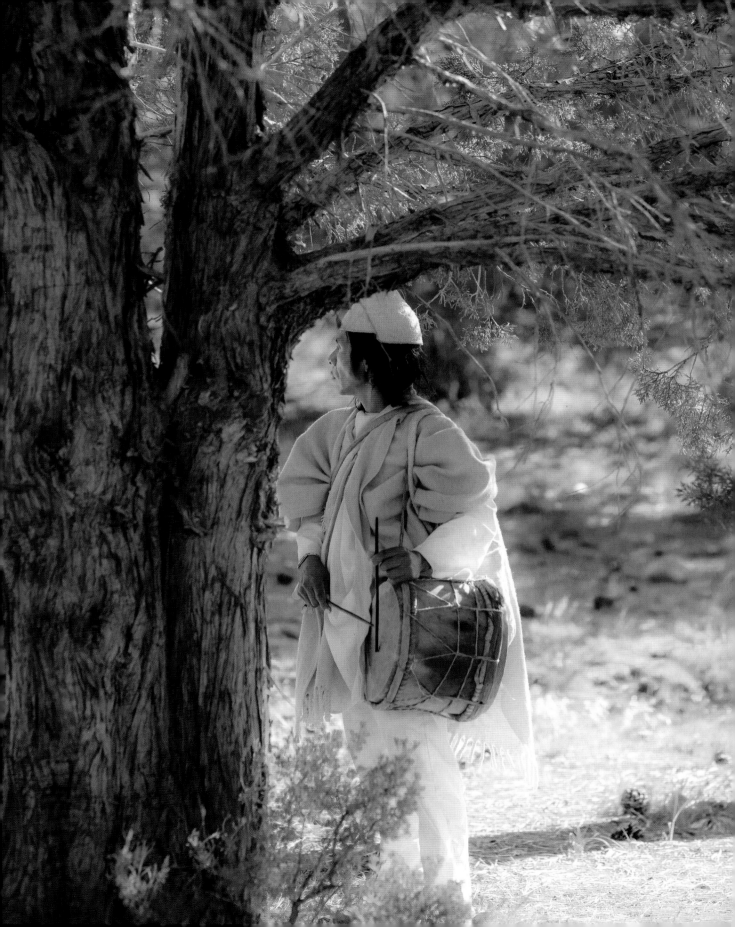

Offering Spirit Plates

Grandmother Clara Soaring Hawk
Ramapough Lenape ✳ United States

*Whenever you sit down to have a meal, it is incumbent upon
everyone to remember their ancestors.*

Meals are also a time for families to come together and this ritual is a remembrance
of this. We both honor our ancestors and acknowledge the importance of life centered
on family values.

We would not be here without our ancestors. It's always good
to honor them. When you sit down, you bless your food. You
serve your plate. Have a small plate on the side. Whatever
you serve yourself, put a little bit on that plate too. I even go
as far as, whenever I'm having something to drink, to put a
small bit in a little copper cup.

The words used for this prayer should come from the
deepest part of your soul. Giving thanks to the ancestors for their sacrifices and service in their lifetime and
for their teachings and protection. Give thanks to those
who have moved on and the spirit of the ancestors who
still remain on the land.

The food is offered as it was life sustaining for
them and us.

When you have finished your meal, take that
little plate outside. I have a tree that I set the plate
near. I don't know who comes to eat the food. I go
back to get the plate in the morning. If I'm away
from home, I still do this. It's always honorable to
remember your ancestors.

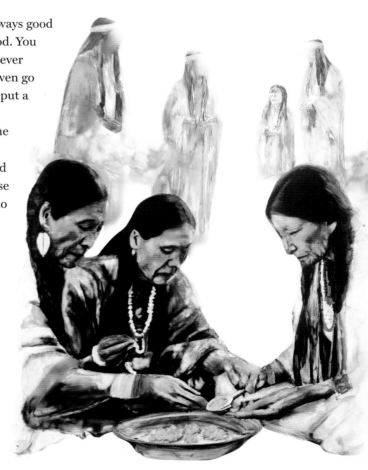

Collecting Stones

Tata Mario Simón Ovalle Chávez
Maya K'iche' ✳ Guatemala

All pebbles are sacred.

When we go on a hill, on a mountain, we take a memory . . . as long as we ask the sacred land for permission to take that energy. That little stone has the essence of the hill. If the hill is powerful for us, then we carry the pebble with us. If you have a pebble from the sea, it has the essence of the sea.

Sometimes, you can buy precious stones, like amethyst, black stone, jade, and quartz, because they protect us. You always have to carry something. Always ask for permission to pick up a stone or anything from nature, even when it's in a shop, because you don't know if the person you are getting the stone from had permission to take it. Because there are also things you cannot take. A person can ask and the land is going to say, "No, not this one."

It depends on what manifestation one feels. For example, grab a little stone on the mountain. Call the spirit of the mountain, the ancestors who also have traveled that mountain. Ask their permission: "I would like to take this little stone that is going to be for me, for my protection." If you grab the stone and it feels like a good feeling, like maybe air or something warm or a positive feeling, it is true. But, sometimes, we grab something and it gives us a chill in our hand or a chill in our body or, suddenly, when we grab the pebble, the image of a person who is not so positive comes to us. That means it is not good. It is not true.

Above all, you have to ask for permission for there to be a response. It comes or it doesn't come. We don't have to carry all things, right? Even from a sacred place.

Cleansing Crystals for Visions

Nana Rosalía Zavala and Ixquik Zavala
Maya K'iche ✶ Guatemala

Cleansing the stones.

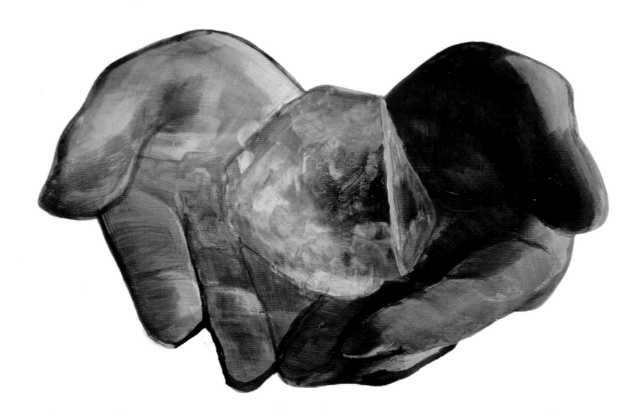

Look for thirteen kinds of plants to place underneath the object, the stone.

Make a mandala to place a stone of any kind in. Place behind it the leaves, seeds, stems, roots, any part of the plant—it's better if they are medicinal.

With your mandala and with your stone, present it to the directions, which also represent the elements and parts of the human body—Spirit of the Air (the breath, North), Spirit of Fire (heart, East), Spirit of Earth (feet, West), Spirit of Water (left and right sides of the body, South), Heart of Heaven (from the navel up, Up), Heart of Mother Earth (from the navel down, Below). I always like presenting in the directions and then placing it.

Leave the stone for 20 days.

It is being cleansed. Everything is healing. The energy from the plants will help heal and purify. This element we are cleansing for ourselves is for vision, something we need clarity on. There are twenty energies, twenty Nahuals (energies for each day of the calendar) integrated in both animals and plants on Mother Earth. That's why we leave it for 20 days. The ancestors will do the cleansing so we can continue our personal healing, our liberation. Through this process we do, of cleansing the stone, we manage to have the vision. Through sleep, it can give us dreams.

For dreams, we use purple quartz. It brings clarity to dreams when there are messages that are obstructed or lack connection. We connect to the dream through wearing quartz. Place it at the forehead and wear it at the heart.

Where does this quartz rest? It has to stay under the pillow so the dreams flow in the connection through sleep. The prayer comes from the heart, the vision through dream, the message of the ancestors from their lineage.

If you do this and don't receive dreams, it still needs light integrated with you and with your quartz. You need to use a candle. This can be done for 7 days, or for 13 too, until the dreams come. It can be done every day. Do 5 sessions minimum, leaving the quartz under your pillow. No compromises. Light the candle. Always use the breath to carry that message from within.

After 5 days, the quartz collects and concentrates the vision, the dream energy that is activated. Put it in water and leave it resting for another 5 days at your altar. Then, you can ask of it. We use it to search for a vocation. What am I here for? What is my mission on Earth? People ask how to know when to be able to conceive. If you are already doing a project or have a job, but feel unsure what it is you have left to accomplish, you can use this process to find the truth. It is a vision quest through purple quartz.

Make the connection. Leave it under your pillow. Then, 5 more days in water, and 5 sessions at the altar. You will have a clear vision.

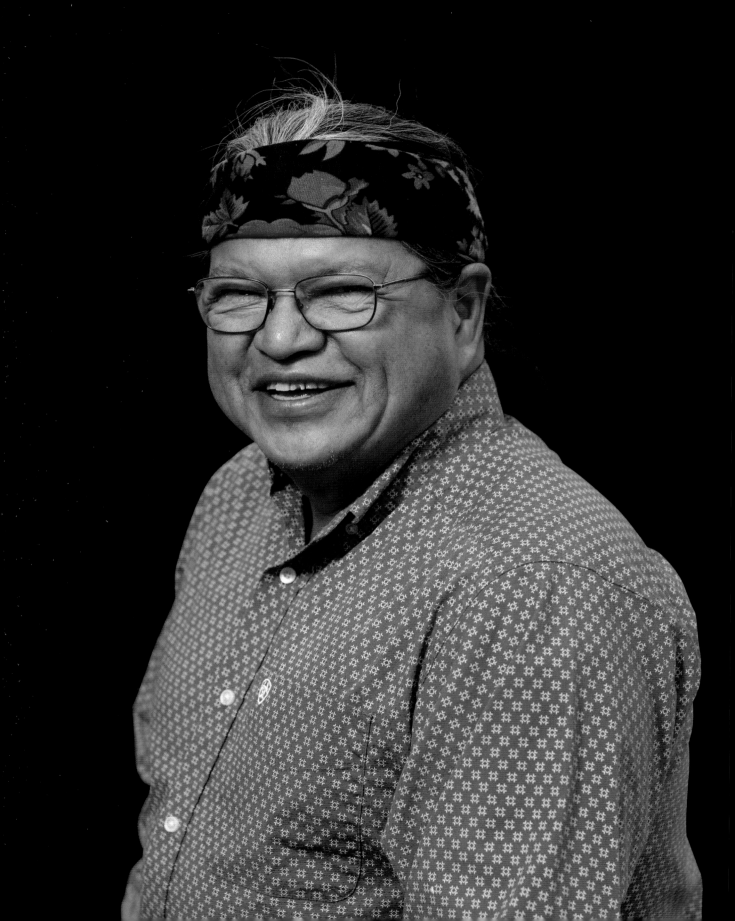

PATRICK SCOTT

Diné (Navajo) ⁂ United States

Patrick Scott is a gifted spiritual leader. He was born and raised in White Mesa, Arizona. Patrick grew up primarily in the government boarding school system and mainly spoke Diné up to his senior year in high school. He began making feather fans while he was still in high school. Upon graduating from Northern Arizona University (NAU) in 1995, he decided to pursue his art full-time. Prior to that, his amazing talent and beautiful creations were well-known only to family and close friends. It didn't take long for his art to become world renowned.

Today, his creations can be found in permanent collections of major museums such as the Gilcrease Museum in Tulsa, Oklahoma; the Smithsonian Museum; Museum of the American Indian in New York City and Washington, DC; Museum of the Plains Indian, in Browning, Montana, as well as galleries and private collections that span the globe. He also makes ceremonial prayer fans used in many Native American ceremonies and feather fans used in powwow and tribal ceremonies. His gourd rattles, staff sets, and drumsticks are valued by the Native American community for use in peyote ceremonies, healing ceremonies, and for other religious purposes.

In traditional Diné ceremonies, Scott followed three different medicine people and learned their ways to become a spiritual leader, hat'aalii, and provide Hozhooji ceremonies, Protection Way ceremonies, Eagle ceremonies, and Blackening ceremonies.

Now, as a husband, father, and grandfather, he is helping his people of White Mesa with all of his heart by building his nonprofit corporation, the Patrick Scott Foundation, a new endeavor for the community of White Mesa.

Body
Opening and Energy

✳

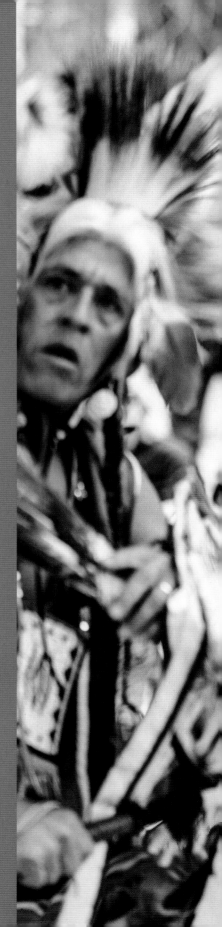

Our bodies are temples. How do you keep the sacred space in the body temple you call yours? Hear from the elders how they regard, maintain, and bless the presence of spirit contained within the human body. Your human vessel might offer more than you think.

———

Notice what and how the elders speak about the body through opening and energy.

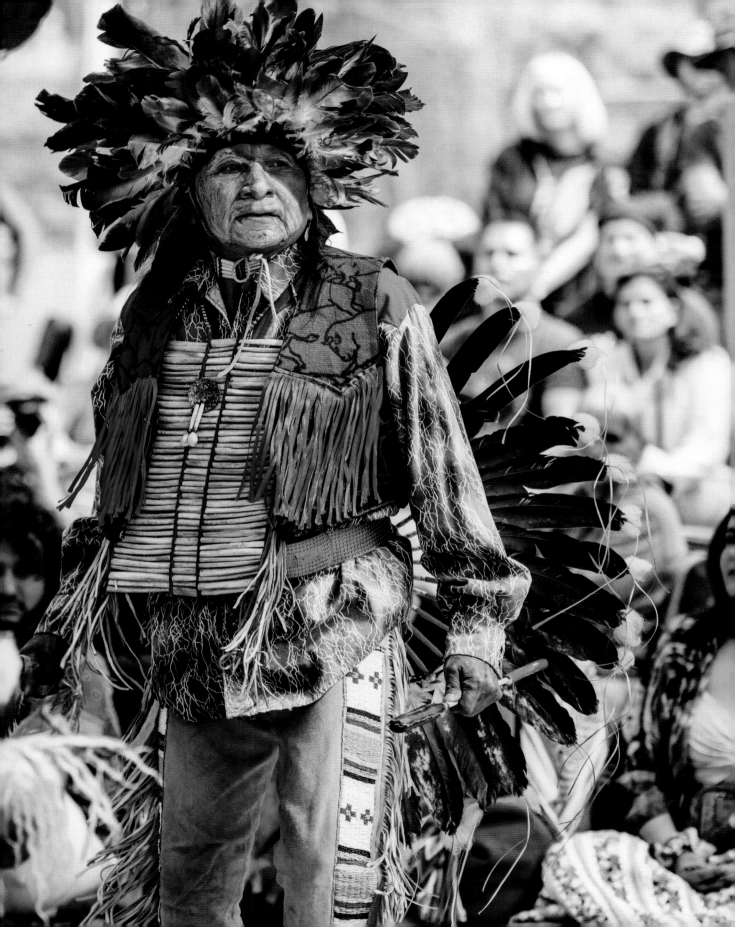

The Four Sources and Codes of Hampi Muju Ruway

Túpaq Ttito Kuntur
Paq'o, Andino ✳ Peru

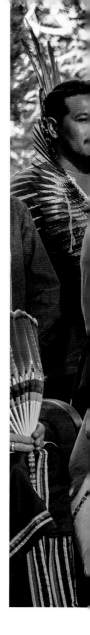

One of the greatest secrets of medicine is that it is within us.
The medicine is within each person.

We don't always have to look outside for healing. We can look within ourselves for our own medicine. We just need to activate it, start a ceremony with it, connect and find the spiritual medicine within us. We need to trust and believe in it. If you don't have faith, the medicine disappears. You have to believe in this medicine and have confidence that this medicine has life, has strength, has power; but for many, it is sometimes difficult to have faith and trust.

It is within us, and outside and beyond so we can connect. There are four sources, four sacred sources of cosmic medicinal power in our bodies. Consider the centers as powers of medicine, to activate and create medicine. I'm not just talking about the chakras you may know, but the most important centers that govern medicinal energy. We here in the Andes know them with their own code: Munay, Yachay, Llank'ay, and Kani.

- ✖ **Yachay** is located in the head; it is the capacity and the center of thought and wisdom.

- ✖ **Munay** is located in the heart; it is the center of the energy of unconditional love and Munay.

- ✖ **Llank'ay** is located in the stomach, solar plexus, or abdomen, and the navel. Llank'ay is also the strength and energy in the physical body.

- ✖ **Kani** is the spirit, power, and other essences of the cosmic being.

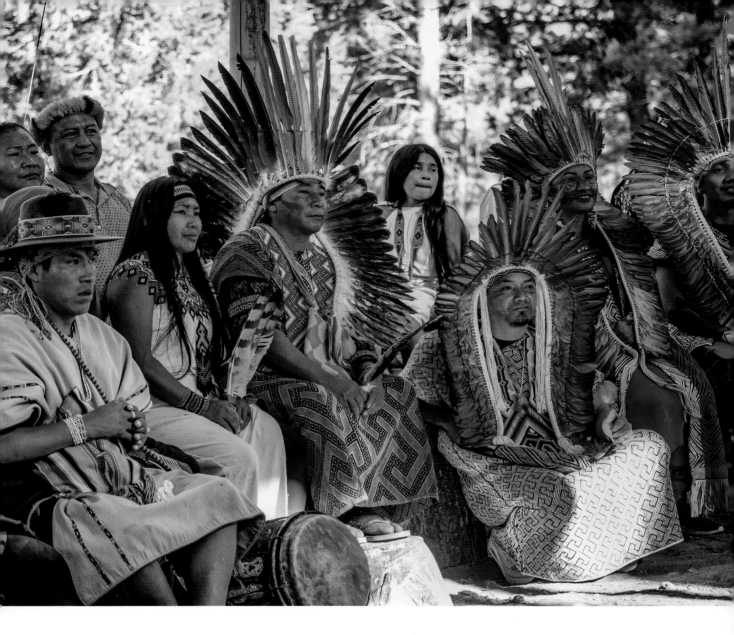

One function of these centers, or sources, is to know, or be aware of, cosmic medicine. These centers have to be connected, synchronized, and in harmony to originate, to give medicine. The code is the knowledge and operation of these centers. The mind has to recognize, to intellectually accept, the cosmic medicine to guide it through the body.

Connecting with the Munay center, with the heart that vibrates, activates cosmic medicine. When we say "heart," we are talking about the physical heart. When we say "Munay," we mean the sacred action of making medicine with the most humble, gentle heart and with unconditional love. That is, by connecting the power of Yachay (mind) with Munay (heart), that is, wisdom with pure and sacred love, we can heal ourselves. We can transmit that energy to our body and heal our illness or free ourselves from those sufferings, illnesses, or conflicts. Munay teaches us to channel. It teaches us to guide and to activate that energy of medicinal love.

If love is not prepared, we have problems, conflicts. We cannot heal ourselves, rather we will hurt ourselves. That love of Munay is a love accompanied by other essences, other medicinal energies born from sources in our body, and is connected with the main source of love, Pachamama.

When I say "Llank'ay," I mean one of the centers that means action—strength to activate cosmic medicine in our being. It is the engine that aims and it is the engine that gives strength to help in the action of medicine with the heart and the mind. This maintains the ability to force and activate medicinal energy.

To heal us, these centers, basically, already have to be connected, synchronized, channeled in harmony and manifesting medicine as the magical colors of the rainbow. Every day we need to be aware of these centers and begin to connect to them.

Kani refers to everything one feels, perceives, and connects—that lives. That is, it refers to what you feel and what you think, what vibrates within you, within your energy, within your cosmic universe, what is all yours. It also refers to all the chakras you know and your deepest self. That's what you are. We have to open, connect, and manifest without fears, without doubts, without emotions, and find the main source of medicine within. It is the spark of light; it is an active force that lives within us, which has different forms and prototypes of energy. It is your own essence, and that essence, that source, that being, no one can change it. That is the medicine to reach the great inner teacher.

Now, there are medicinal pathways and vibrations within you that also manifest in the cells and neurons. Every form of manifestation or medicinal intention in knowledge, in strength, comes from within. We all have to connect with that, with that point through Munay, to activate that necessary energy, that medicinal energy, to heal ourselves and our body.

These centers, these four sources, are like focuses. They look inside and outside of us. They are bridges that interact within our physical dimension, emotional and mental energy, and outward, where the cosmos is, where nature is. So, we have to learn to interact from the depths of ourselves through these centers and from the main source that we say Ñawin of the Khurku Kallpa (meaning the sacred energy centers of the body; "Ñawin" means "eye" in Quechua, referring to these centers being the eyes of our spiritual bodies). We have the Sapan Hampikuy codes for this. (In Inka spirituality every teaching comes with a code, which unlocks dimensions within a person.)

The Codes of Sapan Hampikuy (Personal Self-Healing)

We have to know how to listen to each other, to understand each other. What does your conscience say? What does your mind, your heart say? How can you heal yourself? Or, what is the disease affecting you, attacking you, or bothering you in your body? Take a moment to find or diagnose the illness or disease you have within you. We have to identify the disease to connect with medicine.

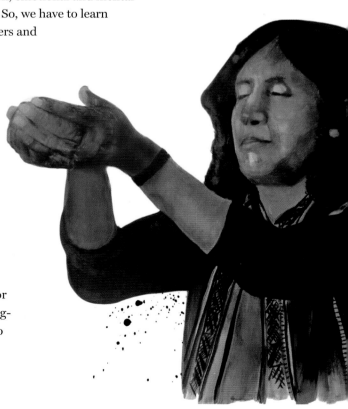

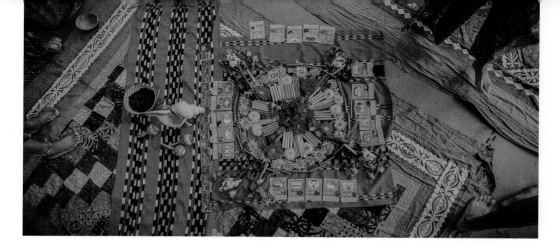

One of the Sapan Hampikuy codes is called Qawaykuy, which means to observe, and observe yourself in detail in a physical and energetic way. Most of the time, either we are very distracted or something distracts us and we do not observe, we do not connect with the medicine. This teaching shows us, directs us, and guides us. How can we put our observation of medicine into practice?

There are two ways to consciously observe: one way is to directly observe everything physical with your physical eyes; but are you really watching?

With the gentlest heart, you are activating your medicinal energy to observe not only with the physical eyes, but to observe with the eyes of energy all forms of medicine, physical and energetic. Put this into practice, whether you are in nature or wherever you are. Put this into practice and you will see the results. Observe with medicinal eyes and heart. With practice, little by little you prepare, connect, and activate your energetic senses for medicinal observation.

When we look, we always find the medicine in some way. Our intention, our vision, has to be to find the true medicine that will help us connect and build on our being. It is not just about observing, but you have to find the point, the secret, where the medicine lives. Where is it in our bodies? In nature? In the plants?

Wherever you go, wherever you are. When you think about medicine, you feel medicine. You want to connect with medicine. Then, it's time to do a small ceremony, as sacred a ceremony as you can that will open the contact and connection with medicine. Get ready, because sometimes the medicinal power of nature and ancestors can surprise you. It may come to heal your energy, or give you a seed so you can help other people.

After doing a small ceremony somewhere, stay there in Ch'innn, in one position, sitting or lying on Pachamama, the Earth, closing your eyes for 1 or 2 hours. This will open and draw medicinal energy into your centers. There, you can connect and build; it is like a flower that blooms and sprouts. This is part of the recognition between your Kani essence and Andean medicine. And so medicine awakens, we call it "Hampi Ruway." It means we are interacting, that we are connecting and building medicinal energy. For this you must have intention, the desire to connect, to heal, to build, and to restore the medicinal energy in your body.

Believe and trust that there is such medicine in the cosmos and seek to connect that medicine. Every moment, every day, we have to look for that connection and maintain that connection. Only then will you stay healthy and strong. Only then will you have the ability to heal yourself and have the medicine in your body. Only then can you feel the medicine inside you.

Cleansing Your Body with Ceremonies

Nana Amalia Tum Xinico

Maya Kaqchiquel ✳ Guatemala

If healing is within the human being by nature, then we must believe that the capacity is within us.

If we believe that our body is sacred, like a sacred temple, then we have the ability to clean it. If people feel some imbalance within them, like they feel chills or they feel very afraid, they feel anxiety or some envy, tell them to grab an egg with the left hand and talk to the egg. It represents a seed that is going to carry everything that happens throughout their body. Rub the egg on the body, then break it in a glass of water and throw it away.

Accompany this with incense. I always recommend using smoke as a partner with the egg to heal, to cleanse, to purify the negative energies. The smoke will also guide you to cleanse your body of any energy it feels.

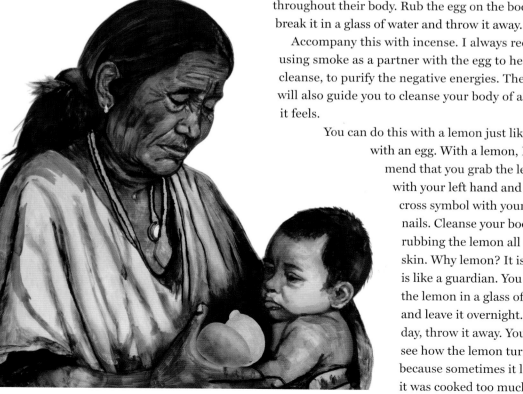

You can do this with a lemon just like you do with an egg. With a lemon, I recommend that you grab the lemon with your left hand and etch a cross symbol with your fingernails. Cleanse your body by rubbing the lemon all over your skin. Why lemon? It is acidic. It is like a guardian. You can put the lemon in a glass of water and leave it overnight. The next day, throw it away. You will also see how the lemon turns out, because sometimes it looks like it was cooked too much and it

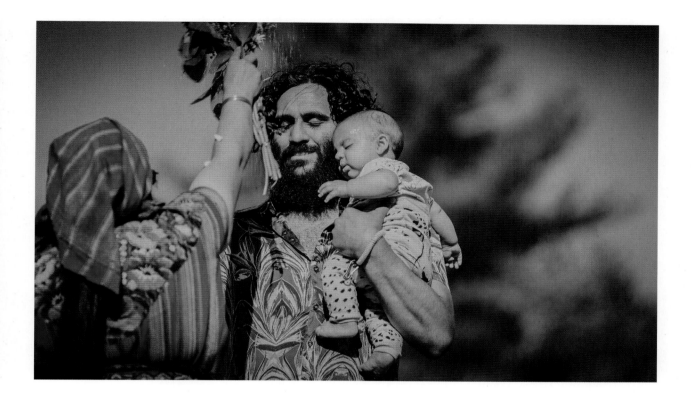

explodes. That means the body has been released through the lemon. The lemon purifies. It unlocks all energy that can be within a person, *as long as this is done with great faith*.

The person has to do this with great faith that they are being freed through this ceremony. Accompany the cleansing with incense or a candle. That is the light. The light must always be maintained because it represents people's inner light. Always do this with the left hand because the left hand unlocks everything in the negative.

For plants, I recommend rosemary and red carnation to cleanse. Here in Guatemala, there is a plant we use specifically for cleansing only, which we call "chilca," but I know you can't find it in other countries. You can use basil; you can use rosemary; you can also use chamomile or the chilca or any flower. Flowers are a symbol of flourishing. Baths with plants are very, very effective. I recommend a bath for 7 days, ready at the moment the person is resting from work.

Boil the plants in water for 10 minutes, let cool, and bathe with it. You have to talk with the water, you have to talk with the plants. A sacred plant that has life, that has essence, talk with it: "Let it purify me, let it cleanse me, let it heal me." Believe that your plants have life, and by connecting with the human being, it frees them from all the tensions, from all the negative energies that people suffer from. When you take the bath, you have that relief, that liberation the next day because you have already cleansed yourself through the bath.

You can do both ceremonies. Use the egg or the lemon on your body to cleanse and heal yourself or make an infusion and then bathe with the water, talking with the essence of the plants.

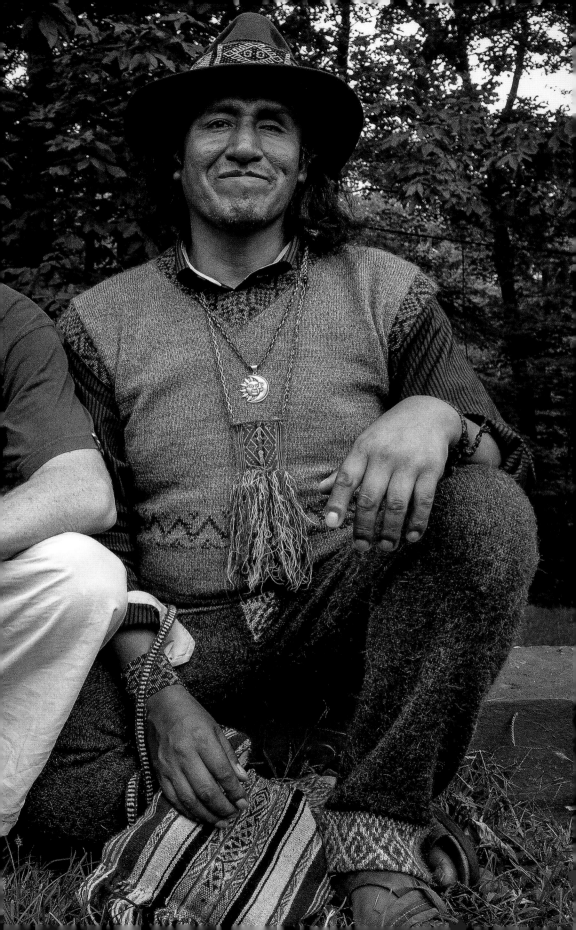

TÚPAQ TTITO KUNTUR

Paq'o Andino, Inka ✴ Peru

Túpaq T'tito Kuntur was born in Cusco, Pomaqanchi, Peru. He descends from pre-Inka and Inka ancestors. His path in Andean medicine continued as a child under the guidance of the Apus (spirits of the high sacred mountains of the Andes), his Inka ancestors, his grandparents, and parents. Túpaq is a spiritual teacher and advisor, guardian of the wisdom and cosmic medicine of the Paqos and Inkas. He is teacher and guardian of the Musuq Tawantinsuyu of the Inkas.

Túpaq has undergone many of the classic initiations to become a Paqo Altomis-ayoq (Acheq Akulleq Paqo), a bridge between the celestial, elemental, and terres-trial realms. He has been struck and confirmed by illapa (lightning) twice—as a child and as an adult—and then, as a teenager, he lost his grandfather and his father tragically too soon. Sick from a mysterious and incurable illness, he left home to learn how to cure himself, thus going through various tests through-out his life. In addition to being in service as Altomisayoq, he has been called to become Willaq Uma (messenger and prophet of the ancestors and the spiritual cosmos of the Tahuantinsuyo of his Inka ancestors), to continue the prophecy left by his ancestors, to reunite and restore the spiritual power of the Tawantinsuyu of the Inkas, along with their brothers chosen for these times according to the Pachakutiq and the Inka prophecy.

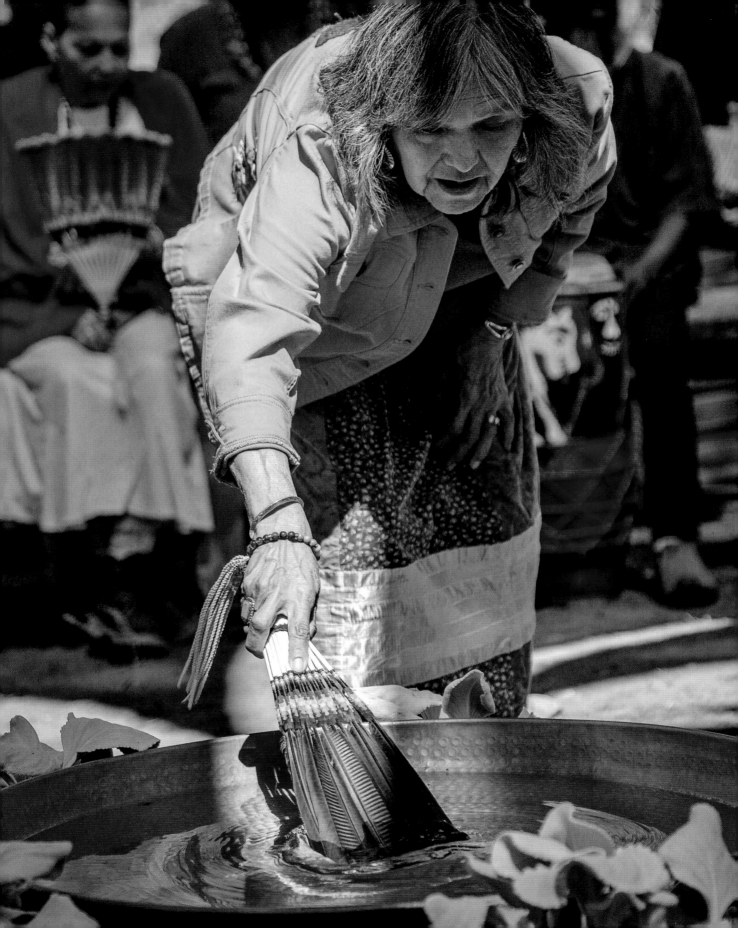

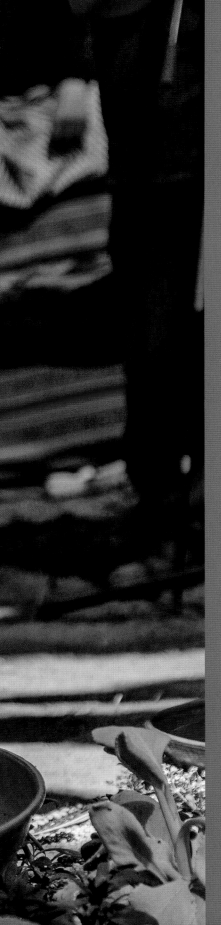

Water

Blood and Ancestors

❋

Water is the current of life. It carries our past through the present and into the future with blessings all must share. Hear from the elders about the importance of being stewards to water and the great responsibilities its greater gifts bring for each of us individually and as generations.

———◆———

Notice what and how the elders speak about water through blood and ancestors.

Giving Thanks to Water

Grandmother Clara Soaring Hawk
Ramapough Lenape ✳ United States

I'm thankful for the water and all the forms she arrives in.

Every morning, I sing the "Water Song." It's a single prayer to give thanks for the water at least once a day. I try to honor the water in every form. The stillness of the ponds. The rush of the waterfalls. The gentleness of snowflakes. The sweet morning dew as it greets each new day.

You know how some days you may feel battered by life and the only way you can feel clean again is to shower or bathe? That is because water is also healing.

I'm thankful for the water and all the forms she arrives in. I'm thankful for the life that she carries and gives. I tell her how sorry I am for the way she was treated. The way she's bottled and sold. Claiming ownership of life-giving and sustaining waters and placing a price tag on her. It's horrible, just terrible; I liken this behavior to slavery. I'm so sorry for these actions and forever thankful that, in spite of the horrible and careless way she is treated, the waters continue to flow.

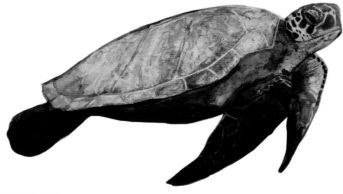

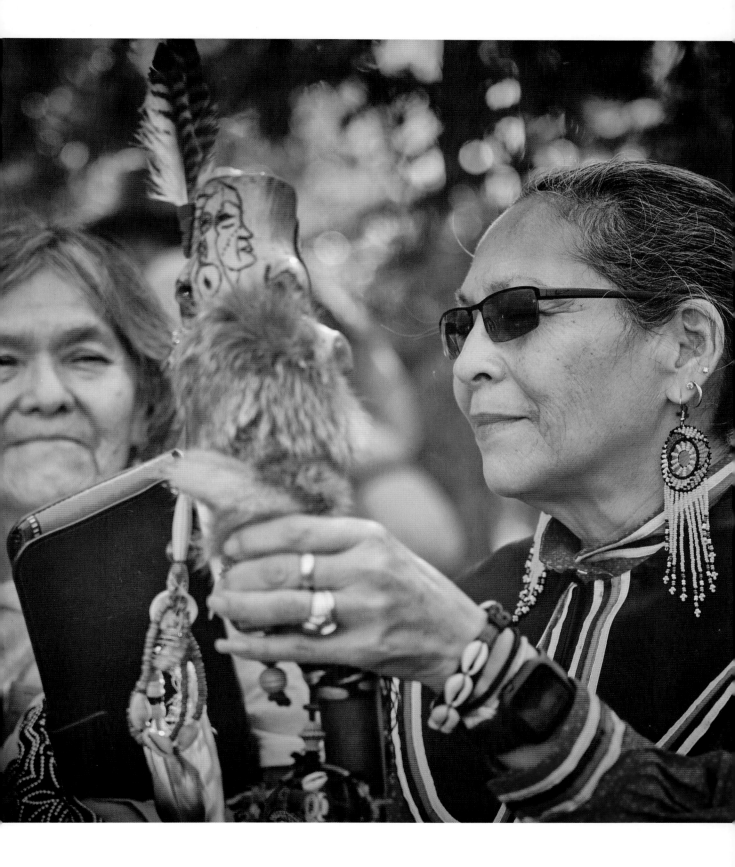

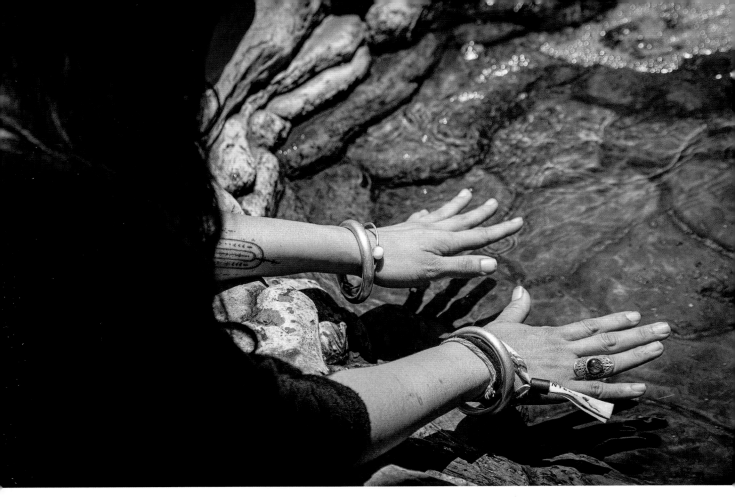

We're created from water. We're carried in water. There has to be balance. Part of taking care of ourselves is to consume a certain amount of water. Our health will deteriorate quickly without water. We can have headaches. So many things can go wrong. It's so important that you know to be thankful. When you have clean drinking water, say thank you. As it's going in your mouth, past your lips and over your tongue, acknowledge that it is going to every organ in your body. It's giving you continued life.

No one should ever, ever, ever take drinking for granted—even a sip of water. It's an honor. It's a privilege that our Earth Mother has given us this water. It's just devastating to see what humankind has done. We all have a responsibility to the water. We are all keepers of the water. We have a responsibility to see that the water is here for the next seven generations and the seven generations beyond that. Our Mother Earth, she's not ours. Never will be. It is our responsibility to care for her now and then turn her care over to our children. That's how it is supposed to go. She's a gift. A gift that's passed forward to the next generation with under-standing. Just like we have a responsibility to care for her now so our children will be able to give her to the next generation. Our children will also bear that responsibility. I don't know when things became so dysfunctional, but we all are keepers of the water and are obligated in one way or another to enact that responsibility.

Hopi Message of Comfort to Say Good-Bye to Loved Ones Who Have Passed

Grandmother Mona Polacca
Hopi, Havasupai, Tewa ❊ United States

This is a message of comfort from the spirit of loved ones who have gone to Spirit World:

I haven't left you. I am here with you.

When you hear the sound of the water bubbling and it makes you smile, that's me.

When you hear the wind blowing and singing through the leaves of the trees, that's me.

*Light a remembrance candle and, when the flame flickers brightly,
that's me giving you the light and warmth of my love.*

Wherever my final resting place is, you know where I am.

I am with you.

Teachings About the Water

Grandmother Mona Polacca
Hopi, Havasupai, Tewa ✳ United States

I come from the water. We all come from the water.

When I was growing up, my mother always told me that her tribe is called the Havasupai, which means "people of the blue-green water." Just by being Havasupai, I am the people of the blue-green water. I've grown up always being told that and that we must always love and respect the water. That we must always pay attention to what is happening to our water. That what happens to water will happen to us.

There is life in water. We come from the water because we lived inside water in our mother's womb. When we came into the world, the water came out before us. We followed it. We are connected through that water. My mother told me that through water we are always connected to our mother. I love looking at pictures of Mother Earth and seeing all that water all around her body. How beautiful it is. We are so blessed to have water, this sacred element.

There are other life forms that depend on the water as well. My mother told me those are our relatives. She would say the fish are our relatives. The plants that grow in the water, they're our relatives. All of life in this world, they are our relatives. She said that when you come into water, you approach it gently. Quietly, respectfully. You walk up to the water and you put your fingers in it. Introduce yourself to it, she said. You introduce yourself by putting your fingers in the water, maybe your toes. Touch it so it receives you and knows you're there. Then, you let it know you're going to swim, enjoy it, or take some of this water back home and use it. Those were the things my mother told me about the water.

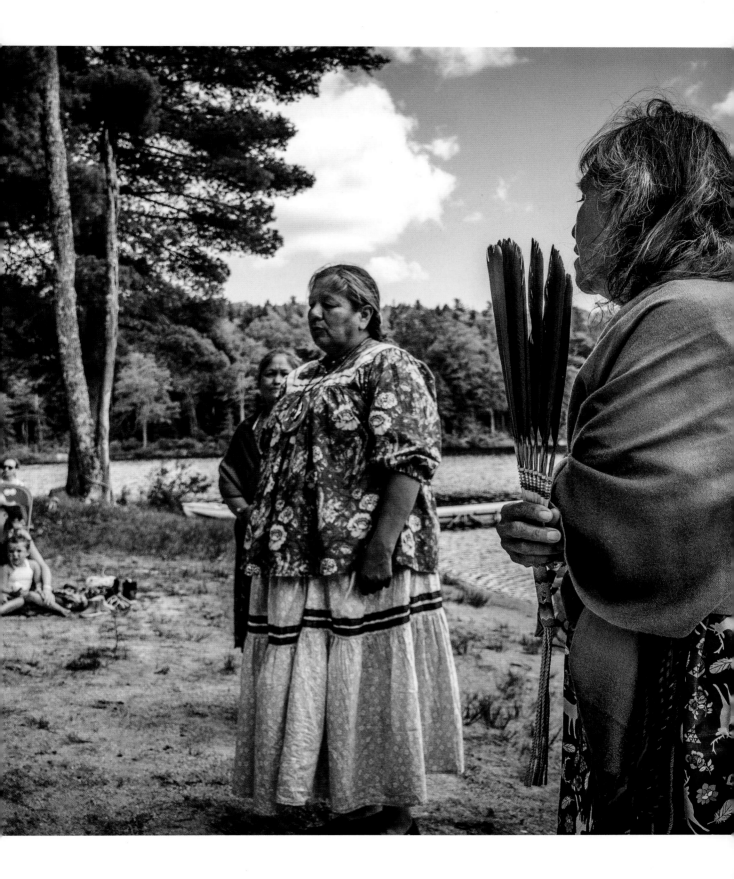

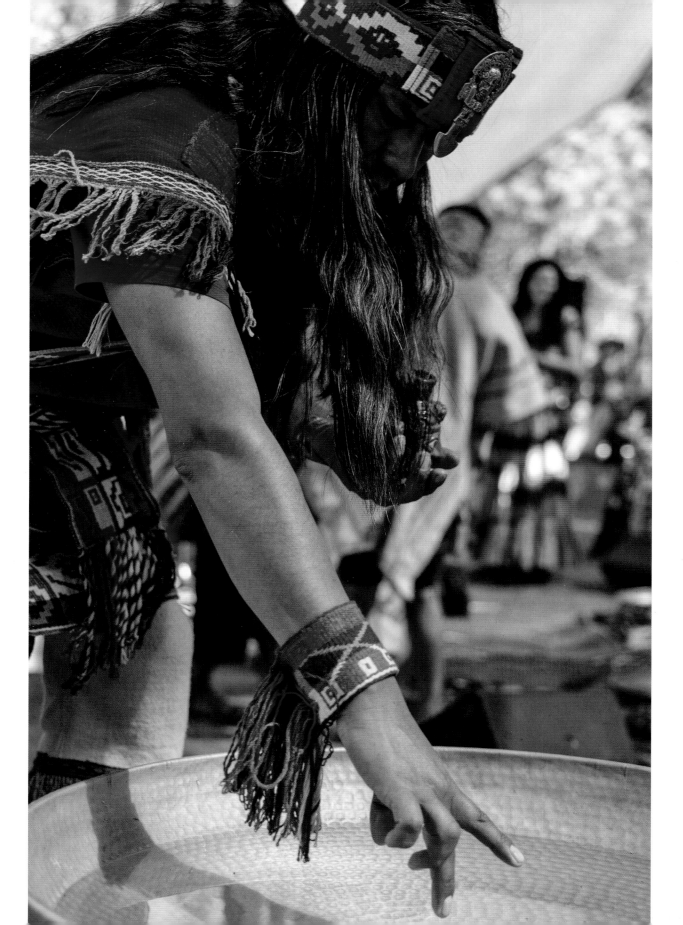

Our family had this custom every Sunday: My mom and my dad would put us children in the car and take us on a drive to the Colorado River. It wasn't that far away from where I was born and raised. We would drive along the river and, at some places, we would stop. We would stop at a place in these little mountains. We would stand there and the river would be far away from us, down below. We'd look at it and how beautiful it was. Then, we would drive some more and would come to a place where there was a beach at the river. We would get out and go to the water. We would do what my mom told us to do: walk up to the water, put our hands in it, call it. We would get used to it, putting our feet and our hands in it before we would go into it. That was part of the teaching, of introducing ourselves to water. We didn't run and jump in—we would gradually go in. You know, you have to be careful and be respectful. There might be a rock and, if you jump in, you get hurt. Come to it gently. We would do that every weekend. Our parents would take us to the water, to the river, and we could see how it was.

On my other side, my Hopi Tewa side, are Pueblo people. They live in high desert lands, where there are no rivers, lakes, or streams. They survive. Part of their survival is from their dependence on their prayers and their ceremonies, done in a cycle of the seasons. That's what they depend on to bring rain, the blessing of rain through their prayers, through their offerings, and through their songs and dances. It requires discipline. It requires being very conscious of their relationship from one generation of the plants, the crops, to the next one. There's no disconnect. When they receive their rain and their gardens grow and they receive the harvest, there are certain preparations they do that are not just having a feast when they harvest, but also in preparation for the coming year. How they prepare their harvest of the corn, the beans, the squash leaves, their plants, their food from their gardens, they prepare it. It's all connected. There's no disconnect from one season to another.

It requires faith. Faith that their prayers are going to be acknowledged and blessed and answered, that they will get rain. Even though there may have been a prediction that there won't be rain or there won't be much rain, they have faith, and they plant anyway because they believe. They have faith that there is a kind, loving, caring, and compassionate Creator that's going to acknowledge them and bring them rain. They continuously follow this pattern. It's their basic survival.

Of all the world religions I have been exposed to, all have a ceremony concerning the blessing water. I've been to the Parliament of the World's Religions. I've been to religious gatherings of all world religions about water. They all have a place where there is a blessing with the water. When it comes to Indigenous People, when we say water is sacred, water is life, it's not something that only we practice. All the world's religions that I know of or have been around use water in a holy manner, just as we Indigenous People do when we say water is life.

I would like to add one more thing about water. This is an honor in memory of a dear, dear friend. He taught that when you go to collect water, you take the water with your container facing downstream, in the direction the water is flowing, and you scoop your water up. That's how you collect your water. You don't take it going in the opposite direction. You take it with the flow of the water. That way it will be good for you. It's all in with the flow of the water we want. Whatever it is we're going to use that water for, it will be used in a good way. Whenever you go to a spring or a place where you collect water, take it in the direction the water is flowing.

Water Ceremony

Túpaq Ttito Kuntur
Paq'o, Andino ☀ Peru

We are going to do a ceremony with a glass of water.

Hold a ceremonial glass of clean water and ask permission to begin the ceremony. Water is conscious and when you talk to it there is interaction, there is communication with the cosmos and with the spirit of that element. So, you have to interact by speaking from your being so you are heard and responded to and connected.

For example, it is like falling in love. When you fall in love with someone, it is something natural. You open your heart between sighs and passion. Something like that has to happen, but in another, more sacred and profound sense where you have to express and communicate.

The water you are working with is sacred. So from this moment on, it is your responsibility what you do with this ceremonial water. Observe the water with your eyes of medicinal energy, with your medicinal heart. It's alive. It is active.

Feel your connection. Believe in her.

This water came to your house, to your hands for this ceremony. Perhaps you have not been appreciating and valuing this water, but now is the time to connect with it and appreciate this water that is alive, that has cells, that is the blood of our Pachamama, of the Apus spirits. This water feels what you are now feeling, thinking, and it is time for you to ask for the medicine of Unu Mama (water). This is how you will receive the medicine.

Remember, you have to trust and have faith in the spirit of water. This sacred and conscious water brings with it a whole mystery. It has walked through the veins, through the channels of the plants, the trees, the Earth, the Pachamama, the mountains, and the streams. It was in the blood of your ancestors and now it is here. This water is present and connected with medicinal spirits.

For this moment of the water ceremony, open your heart and your sacred centers to this moment. Breathe deeply and begin to connect with those centers Munay, Yachay, Llank'ay, and Kani to align your energy, harmonize, and open them. This is a great, sacred time to drink this water medicine.

- Begin by invoking (Pachamama, Mother Earth, Pachataita, Cosmic Father, and spirits and places you feel connected to) and expressing your full name and the energy of your heart from deep within. Connect with medicinal spirits.

- Ask the divine light of the Inka ancestors and the cosmic beings to authorize you and give you this medicine in the water you are going to drink.

- Close your eyes and begin to invoke, 5 minutes, more or less. Do it with patience and tranquility for connection and within you. You must continue opening your channels and preparing your conscious energy to receive this great medicine for the healing of your being or some center.

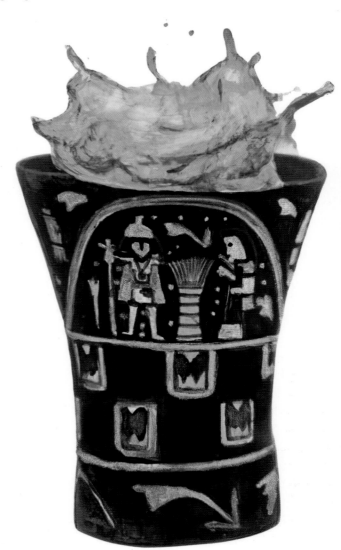

- When you are ready, you can drink and receive the sacred water into your being. Then, you can let the water flow until it reaches the main source of your being for about another 5 minutes.

- At the end of the water ceremony, dedicate a sacred song or melody out of gratitude.

  Medicines as they are had to arrive here with the blessing of the beings, according to our invocation, for this sacred moment of ceremony from the farthest reaches of other dimensions, taking and transcending the paths we call "channels of Seqes," or in other mysterious ways to connect, heal, and help us.

Water Healing for Tormented Minds

Nana Amalia Tum Xinico
Maya Kaqchiquel ✳ Guatemala

The river never returns.

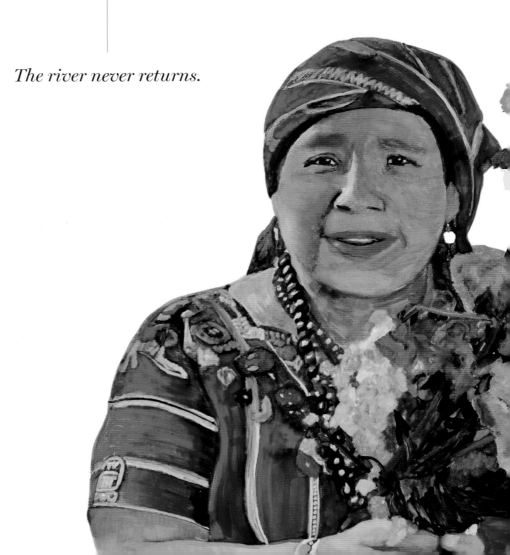

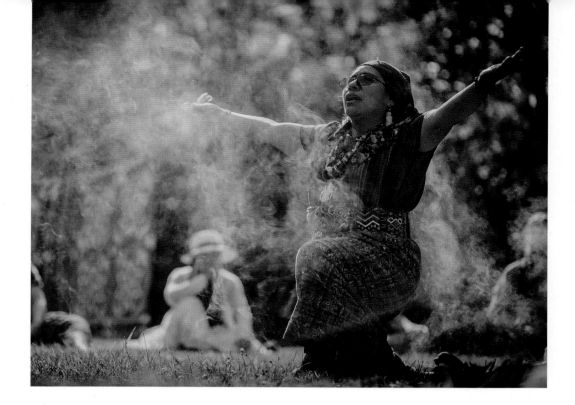

The water flows even though there are so many stones, even though there are so many stumbles.

Water always finds its way and flows.

The human being must learn from water; to flow, to not stay stuck with the feelings that exist, to throw away all those thoughts that no longer serve.

The river teaches us.

Within the Maya culture, there are many tools and ways to heal. I recommend that people heal with water. When there is pain, when there are feelings affecting your mind, it is because the brain comes from water. It is born from water.

You can do a ceremony, not every day.

Write down all of your feelings, all of your emotions.

What are the things you no longer want to have? What are the thoughts that should no longer be here, that don't belong to you? If there are also issues you have been generating from your lineage, simply say, "Thank you, Mom; thank you, Dad, thank you brother, thank you ancestors, but, today, I want to make my life. I want all that does not correspond to me to be cut. I want to do what belongs to me, do what I like, do what I feel in my heart."

Write it on paper. Blow on this paper three times and leave it in the river.

Let everything happen through the water. Water is life. Water is light. Water cleans. Water purifies. It removes all the energies that are bothering you at once, regardless of the space where you are when you find the water.

Find your water and float.

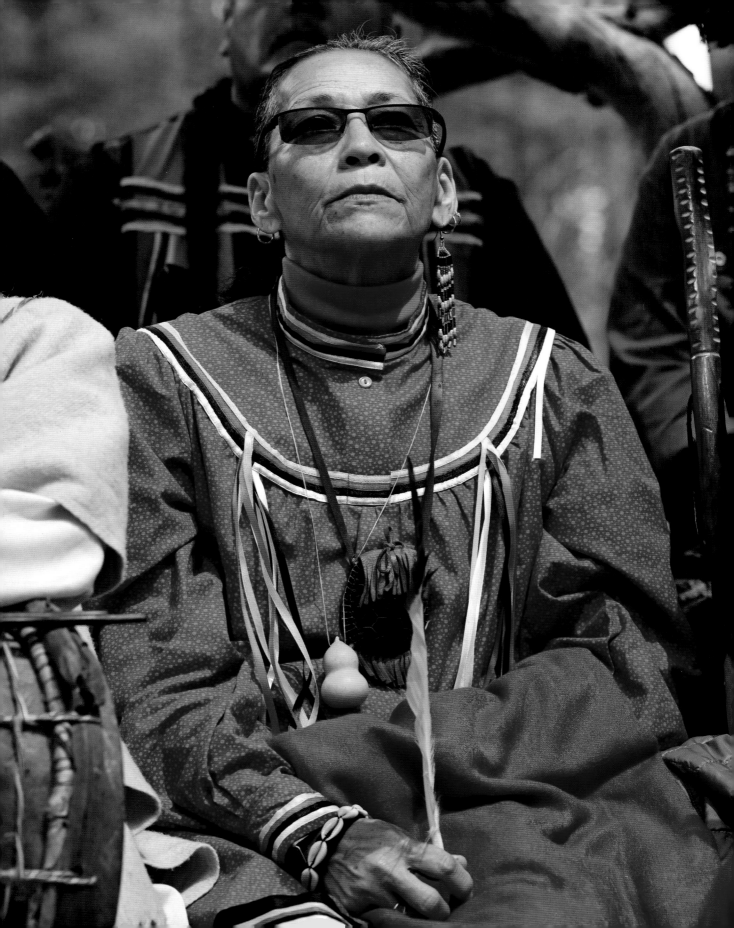

GRANDMOTHER CLARA SOARING HAWK

Ramapough Lenape ⁑ United States

Grandmother Clara Soaring Hawk is a former chief and presently Ramapough Lenape Nation ambassador.

An elder, spiritual advisor, public speaker, artist, activist, and teacher of all truths as they are received from the Creator and the ancestors, Grandmother Clara facilitates ceremonies both nationally and internationally at a multitude of events and spiritual gatherings. She supports and takes an active role working with the youth.

Grandmother Clara defines herself as a spiritual ecologist. "In this time of global turmoil, we must be open to a new level of consciousness.

"I stand for the water. I stand for the land. I stand for the people. I *rise* for the next seven generations!"

Kliloona Lunaapeewak—we are all one people.

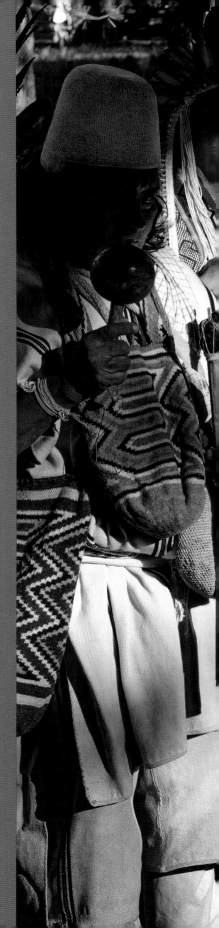

Clearing
Release and Healing

✳

Clearing makes way for the sacred. It is an emptying of vessels for the power of creation to come in as it must in this moment. Letting go of the past is the first act of creation in the present. Hear from the elders about how they practice ceremonies of clearing to aid in aligning our thoughts, feelings, and actions with the call of whatever the present unfolding brings.

———

Notice what and how the elders speak about clearing through release and healing.

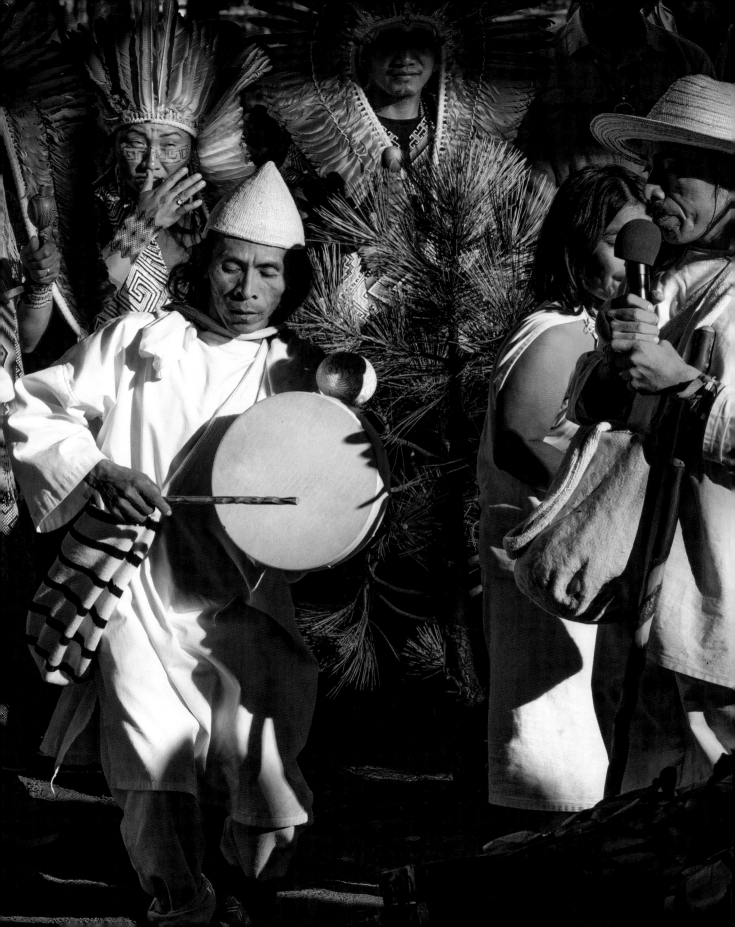

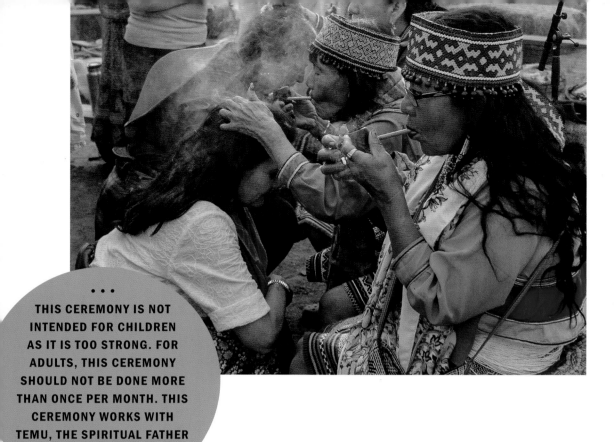

Deep Energy Clearing and Reset

Rodrigo Kakamukwa

Mamo Wiwa ✳ Sierra Nevada of Santa Marta, Colombia

These two consecutive baths may be done at night to do a total reset of your energy field, particularly to clear some residual foreign energies. Take a bath with this recipe on two consecutive nights.

Don't use aged rum that has a golden color. It has to be clear rum, and it has to be rum because rum is alcohol made from sugarcane and that is the Spiritual Father in nature who will be helping you.

There are two species of eucalyptus: one with smaller, rounded leaves and the other with bigger, elongated leaves. Use 9 leaves if they are rounded and small, or 9 pieces of eucalyptus leaf if the leaves are bigger and elongated.

Bath instructions

BATH MATERIALS

9 lime leaves (not lemon)

9 eucalyptus leaves

8⅓ cups (2 L) clear rum

Put the 9 lime leaves and 9 eucalyptus leaves inside the bottle of rum. Wait at least 4 hours for the leaves to infuse the rum (I do this the night before).

The first night you take the bath, use half of the rum, lime, eucalyptus mixture (4 cups plus 2½ tablespoons, or 1 L, of the concoction plus 1 bucket, any size, of water). Put the rum in the water and mix it a little.

You need a small cup to use to pour the water on your body—you will wash your entire body with it. While washing with the water, ask the Spiritual Fathers in nature, including your guides and Jose Maria Kakamukua, to help you remove from your aura/energy field the dark energies of Temu (Spiritual Father of darkness) as well as the red energies of Temu and the transparent energies of Temu.

Wash your back, arms, legs, and hips well.

For your chest, wet a washcloth with the water and alcohol to clean your chest. Do not clean the nipples.

For your face, use the washcloth wetted with the water and alcohol mix to clean your forehead (third eye), temples, base of the skull, neck (back and front), and put a little bit of the liquid on your crown, always with the intention to clear those energies (witchcraft).

Pay close attention to your back and the shoulder blades—if you need to use more of the mixture, do it. **Do not rinse your body with water**.

Dry your body with a towel lightly; dry your chest well. Put on your pajamas, perform two full body rotations counterclockwise, and go to bed.

The next morning, take a shower as you usually do with soap and water. That day, at night, repeat the exact procedure with the remaining 4 cups plus 2½ tablespoons (1 L) of the alcohol and leaves mixture. Do not forget to make the two full body rotations counterclockwise after the second alcohol bath. The following morning, take a shower as usual.

What the Sweat Lodge Represents

Patrick Scott
Diné (Navajo) ✳ United States

The sweat lodge is made of tree branches.

You sit in the center, then the whole thing is covered with mud. It's like going back into the mother's womb and then back into childhood, into that stage of innocence when there were no rules, no protocols for the way to live. There was no distortion. There was nothing. You were just part of nature.

Getting back to that stage opens your thinking in different ways. When the heated rocks are brought to the sweat lodge, that opens the pores throughout your body. On that deeper level, on the inside, the process brings up a lot of things (emotional, mental, physical, and spiritual healing).

The sweat lodge takes you to another, deep level. The process starts removing a lot of stuff in your body that doesn't belong there. Then, by adding more hot rocks and pouring more water over them, the sweat lodge is made very, very hot; very intense. There are two purposes for this: to get the really deep stuff inside of you out of your system and to open your pores and just kind of breathe. That's what sweat lodge is intended to do. You sweat really fast to open your pores. It cleanses your body.

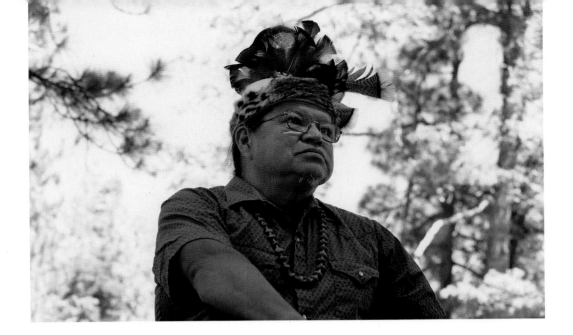

You just close your eyes and don't say anything. Nobody says a word. You just sit through the whole thing for 10 minutes at 180°F (82°C). Sit there and meditate. Just purely meditating. That calms your mind, calms your body, and then challenges you into that intense heat. It's there, but you challenge your body to shut the whole thing off; shut the system off and get into a calm state and sit there to meditate. This is a practice we do all the time.

This is a way of calming the brain, calming the body, and having the blood flow from your heart out—away from the heart. Then, once I get out of the sweat lodge, I usually go into a very cold place that shuts down the body's pores really fast. In winter, I lie in the snow. When you do that, it constricts and brings all the blood back to your heart.

Those are the basic things we do in sweat lodges. Culturally, it gets more complicated. We use sweat lodges to socialize. All the men come together and they tell each other about whatever is going on in their lives. This is integrated into sweat lodge. It's a good place to come together and connect with each other.

Another part of sweat lodge is to share our songs, to learn our songs and the prayers for them. Those practices we do, maybe, twice a week if we want to learn some of these ways. We go there and we sing, we sing, we sing and we explain the songs. We talk about the songs, about the prayers—what they mean and how we use them. Then, we get into the real details of a lot of these ceremonies. What songs can we sing when we travel? We have hunters who have special ceremonies to go out hunting. They put different songs on themselves to help them connect and make their centers really sensitive. The tiniest movement of animals, they can sense these things. They put themselves in the sweat and put those songs on themselves. Then, they have to go back to the sweat lodge to remove that energy they put on before going back into the community.

We have 9-day ceremonies. After we finish the whole ceremony, the people who participated can't just go back into the public with all that energy on us. So, we have sweat lodges. We take this energy off before we go back to work or home. It gets very complicated trying to explain. There's quite a bit involved. These are very old, old practices.

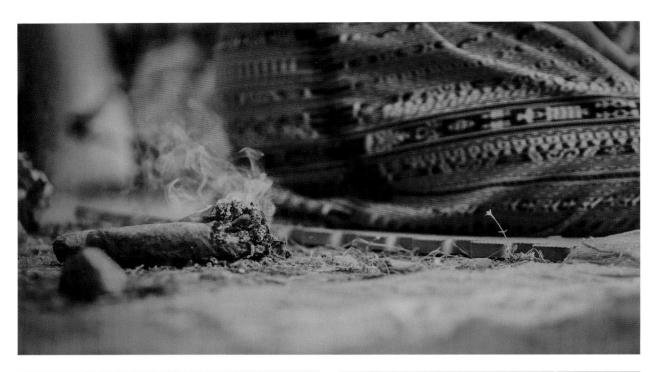

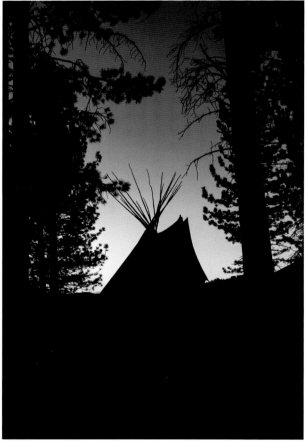

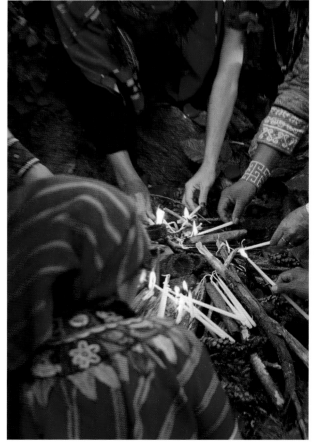

Cleansing Ceremonies

Nana Rosalía Zavala and Ixquik Zavala
Maya K'iche ✴ Guatemala

There are four elements important in the Maya worldview that we make various forms of connection with.

The first is the *energy of the wind*, which is our breath because air is the first element we breathe when we are born. It is our first contact where our energy activates like the lungs of the universe and the lungs of Mother Earth. We internalize this in our body. That's why we start with the element of air. When we talk about the element of air, we use breathing as an element in spirituality like food. We use plants, incense, copal, flowers. We always inhale it as a sign of the first connection of air. You inhale deeply. You can do it 3 times or up to 20 times. The air element connects. Inhale. Exhale.

The second element, *fire*, concentrates our hand energy. In that connection, we understand that the heart is the first organ formed when life is created at our conception and, therefore, is the second moment that connects us: the moment that activates our hands, when we have the opportunity to open them when we are born. It is clear that this energy of fire is always present in the energy of our hands. It materializes through an offering of a candle. We keep a light in our house, in our space, to always keep in mind the knowledge of the heart. We unite that energy of fire in our hands. We have a word, "maltyoox." It is our ancestor's way of saying the breath or sigh of the heart that comes from within. When we learn to pronounce this word, we feel that heat coming out from within. Listen to that heartbeat, that thought.

We connect with the third element, the *Earth*, through a copal tree. It could be an incense burner. It may be a plant we have to connect to the energy of Mother Earth. We keep aromatic plants that we can dehydrate present on our altar. We have this in our space. We can put it on the ground, under a tree, under a flower that takes our intention into the ground. It is the way our material body carries an energy transmission to the body of Mother Earth in a spiritual way.

The fourth element we have is our *connection with water*. Liquid can reach our body and activate what flows in our body. We talk about the internal waters of our body. Here, we have another way of connecting water. From the internal cleansing of our waters to the external cleansing of Mother Earth with the support of the mineral kingdom. We use a quartz or an obsidian of various shapes. When we want to make an internal cleansing of our waters, we use the element of water along with any minerals that center and integrate our body. The integration happens from within.

This enters into processes of trauma, family, and social problems. Obsidian is used more with the integration of the element of water when there are sexual traumas. We use obsidian for a reason—because this is a materialized element of the pain of Mother Earth and of the great volcanoes that produce liberation. Just as Mother Earth's body releases, we use this element to free ourselves. In this way, we use these elements of the mineral kingdom externally because we understand that, on Mother Earth, there are ways in which the ancestors came to connect with the spiritual world from the outside.

When we talk about sexual trauma, we can talk about whether it is from a relationship or whether from childhood. There is a process when these things happened in childhood. For this, we use an obsidian egg because the energy of the child has not yet opened to life. There is no sexual consciousness in their world. That's why the obsidian is an egg. We place the obsidian in the navel so you can reconnect with your spiritual being and do the internal clearing and healing according to your genital parts, then we put the obsidian egg in water overnight to purify that energy. We drink the water in the morning to cleanse internally. If the sexual trauma happened in youth or adolescence or adulthood, the obsidian is placed at the heart, then left in water overnight, and the water is drunk in the morning. Truth in the heart. This is what is achieved with the obsidian: We create transformation of what has passed and bring it back to life in a way of harmony.

We use white or rose quartz if the trauma is in a relationship, if someone has been used or subjected to abuse, whether the man or the woman. You integrate the quartz into the water, leave it overnight, and then drink the quartz water. It is taken the next day, in the morning with the ray of the sun so it continues doing the cleansing. If this is a couple in a relationship, the water is not drunk. It is settled under a tree or a plant. Any plant. It can be medicinal or a fruit tree.

All these processes are done for 7 consecutive days. Seven days. We talk about 7 days because there are 7 ways of understanding pain. That's why we do this for 7 days in a row to do the cleansing.

With this cleansing, you need to do a piece of writing. You need to write 20 positive intentions, personal desires, and 20 ways you have felt that pain materialize as an object of trauma and that you wish to cleanse. How have you felt it? Twenty positive things. Twenty negative things. Write all this down, put it on your altar or a space where you will read it again—every

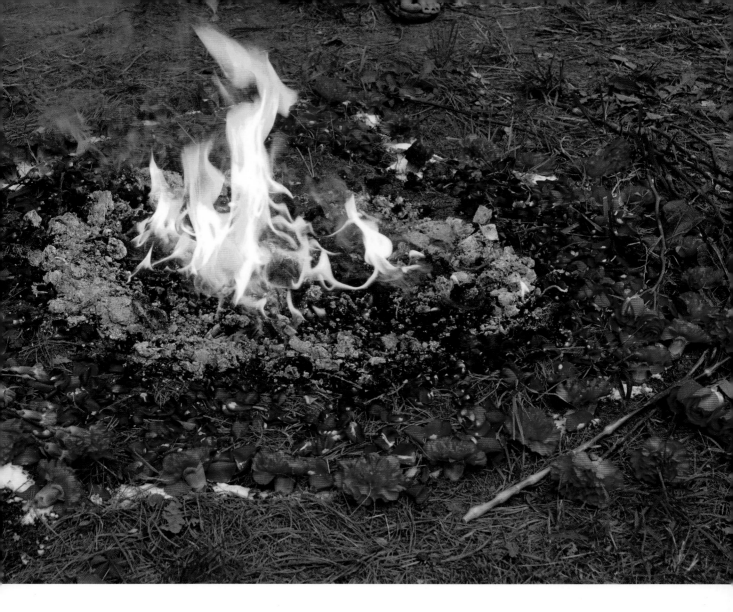

moment, the good and the bad. Every day, read for 7 days. Every day you reread it. That's how we look for duality, that balance. The good is part of the bad and the bad is part of the good. In that balance, you learn how to face it and be able to see it another way.

After 7 days, burn it. Offer it to the energy of good. Blow it, leave it, deliver it to nature, and keep processing, keep releasing the trauma and situations.

Let your emotions be released however they need to be—screams, cries, with a hug, with an instrument or drum. Let it go free with whatever sound supports it. Sometimes, there's a disconnection between the material and the spiritual body. The truth is, some sound can help keep it in balance.

If you need to do it all again, you can leave 13 days in between for the spirit to go. You need that transition from time to time. Then, 7 days and 13 days of intermission, as many times as you need it. You can repeat until you feel you are emptied.

The point of balance is when you feel there is nothing more to release.

Wisdom of the Kava

Papali'i Dr. Tusi Avegalio
Polynesia ⁂ Oceania

Curing is removing all evidence of disease.

Healing is to make whole again. One can be cured but not healed.

The Kava Ceremony

Throughout the region, the kava ceremony has been part of ceremonial occasions since ancient times. The installation of traditional titles, agreements between villages, the welcoming of an important visitor, or rendering high respect by hosts will always include a kava ceremony. In Tonga, Fiji, and Sāmoa, the installment of kings or noble titles is not complete without a kava ceremony. In the same token, kava ceremonies assuage harmful divisions, acts of violence, and can even end war with the kava's mana (elemental power) of healing and forgiveness.

This kava cultural history has many applications in life. Among many modern societies, reductionist thinking sees the parts that make up the whole. Hence, regarding health treatments, the emphasis is on curing. On the contrary, Polynesian societies see the whole that organizes the parts. Hence, in our traditional ceremonies and protocols the emphasis is on healing.

Curing and healing are not the same thing. Curing removes all evidence of disease. Healing makes one whole again. One can be cured but not healed. The symbolic meaning of the circle of the kava bowl connotes the whole, and the kava the substance of healing.

The application of this wisdom is particularly poignant in traditional protocols of respect and leadership. The kava ceremony is the highest form of respect in Polynesia (Sāmoa, Fiji, Tonga, Rarotonga), Melanesia (Fiji, Vanuatu), and Micronesia (Pohnpei, Kosrae). Its integrity is enhanced with the presence of respected elders with genealogical ties, cultural wisdom, language/oratorical capacity, traditional tattoos, and rank status.

Kava wisdom for leaders is: Good leaders lead. Great leaders heal.

Salient examples of great leaders in history are Martin Luther King and Abraham Lincoln of the United States, Nelson Mandela of South Africa, Mahatma Gandhi and Mother Theresa of Indian fame, Hin-mah-too-yah-lat-kekt Chief Joseph of the Nez Perce, Queen Lili'uokalani of Hawai'i, and Tupua Tamasese Lealofi III of Sāmoa. Sadly, history also shows that there are times when one must bleed to heal when peaceful resistance is disregarded. Please add to this list by sharing those of your culture or nation.

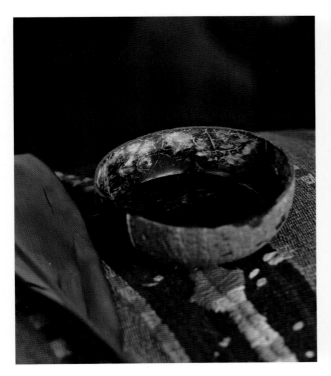
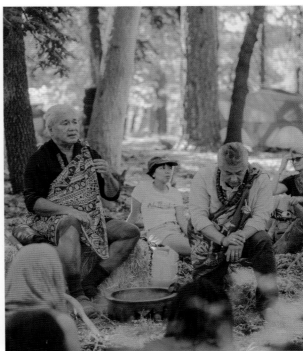

Kava Origin Story

Kava's origins are from the Manu'a Islands of the Sāmoan archipelago (though kava origin stories vary throughout Oceania, the common root theme is bringing together through healing).

A high priest in ancient Sāmoa had a son who consumed the food offerings to Tagaloa (god of the universe). In god-like wrath, Tagaloa split the son in half with a lightning bolt—from head to groin. Moved by the grief of his faithful high priest, Tagaloa directed him to a special plant to obtain its roots, crushing them and mixing the crushed roots with water. A carved wooden bowl was then filled with the mixture. Tagaloa sent a gentle rain to add to the mixture. Tagaloa then instructed the high priest to hold the parts together and pour the mixture between the split seam of his dead son, and utter "Manuia" (good health, to prosper, be happy). Tagaloa then responded with "Soifua," or long life. At this pronouncement, the separate parts of the boy healed and he was made whole again with life, and the boy sat up alive. The high priest clapped his hands in joy. Thus are the origins of kava and the significance of the sacred wooden container, the kava bowl. With the admonition that kava pertains to high chiefs and is sacred, Tagaloa took his leave.

Kava Serving, Receiving, and Drinking Protocol

Ceremonies since that day involve the receiving of the ipu (half-shell coconut cup). When your name is called, clap your hands. The server will then approach you with an ipu of kava. First, offer a few sprinkles to the gods, a small speech appropriate to the occasion, drink the kava, and end with the word "Manuia." Those gathered respond back with "Soifua."

Clearing Ceremonies for Travel and Home

Tata Mario Simón Ovalle Chávez
Maya K'iche ✳ Guatemala

When you come home, at the time of entering your house,
you always need the elements.

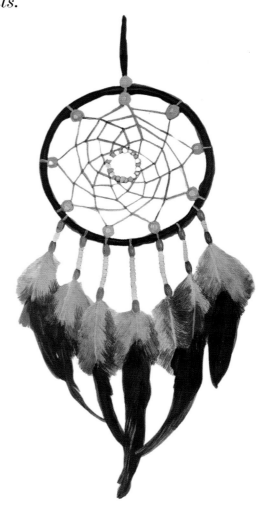

Outside, there are many strong energies, whether from the environment, from the people, or from the spaces you go, that have an impact. So, it is highly recommended to have some sacred smoke at the door where you enter. Light it and smudge yourself with the smoke, then enter. That helps cut off the strong energies or negative energies one often picks up from the places you've been.

Our bedrooms are our places of rest. Sometimes, energies, bad thoughts, and all that can leak in because it's our place of rest. Try to make sure it is clean. Many times, I have experienced things that are not appropriate appear in the space. People say they have an animal under their bed or they heard a sound. So, we do a purification. Purify, purify, always purify the spaces. Purify oneself.

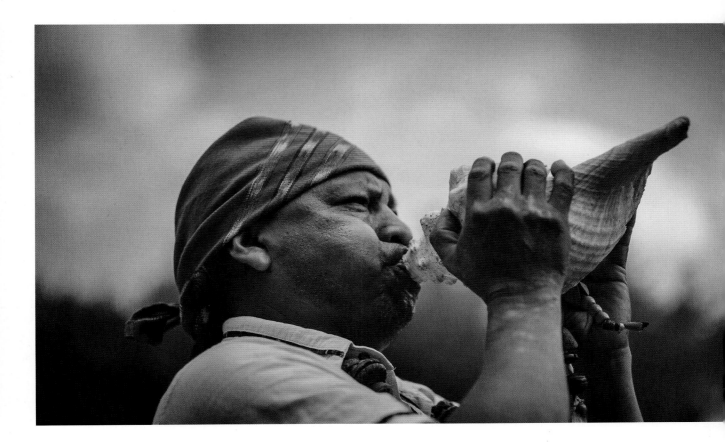

Likewise, let's say you go to an event. This can be spiritual too. They provide you with a chair to sit in, for example. Normally, what you have to do there is to bring at least a handkerchief or a paper napkin or whatever and rub that chair. Like cleansing, cleansing, cleansing. It doesn't matter that it is already very clean, but you have to clean it because people sit and leave their energy there. In a public place or a place where there are a lot of people you don't know. That's why we always say you have to smudge everything you have in a house. Many times, that cannot be done, so this cleansing is a symbol of sweeping away, of bringing out truth in that place where you are going to be when you are away from home.

This is a ceremony to cut off the energy that was there before you, because sometimes it can catch you. If there is energy there, you may get a headache, you may feel unwell. To be calm, you have to do the sweeping, symbol of cleansing, and then sit down. This works very well anywhere in any space. In a car, even on a plane. Treat it symbolically because that's what we're doing—cleansing as a ceremony.

Let's say you are going to be somewhere for a while. Internally, ask the ancestors that everything in the space be cleansed, to let it not be contaminated. Perhaps in the case of many people abroad in both Europe and the United States who travel a lot, when they go to a hotel or any house where they stay, maybe they bring small incense and smudge the space. A little bit on the bed, a little bit of the space. Sometimes, the smoke is not allowed. Bring a piece of paper or a napkin and clean because, sometimes, those spaces are very contaminated.

It is good to do this clearing with prayers.

If you have a healing mission and someone comes along asking you to purify them, you will need either plants or candles or tobacco or water or a stone. Many times, there are very strong energies and there is a need for, let's say, a quartz stone. You have to have it. If you have to cleanse a person and you feel the energy is very strong, you can do cleanse, that purification. Quartz or obsidian is very powerful. You just wash it well with water and blow sacred tobacco or copal smoke over it so it recovers and releases that person's energy.

You can use obsidian to cleanse yourself or another person. Pass it around your energy body, your hands, feet, everything. The whole body. Do it slowly with your prayers. Contact with the skin heals better.

When you buy your vehicle, it is very important to do this ceremony. It doesn't matter if it's new. Did you ask for cleansing and for protection when you purchased it? Even when someone bought my car, we opened it, opened the hood, and we passed candles and incense underneath everything so it doesn't fail, so there are no accidents or crashes. People feel very good. They feel very protected.

Use sacred incense or candles and do a prayer of protection and gratitude. A vehicle also has its essence. Unfortunately, many people have lost their lives in an accident with their car. That is what we do not want. If we buy a vehicle, it is to help us, to transport us so we can do our work. So many people ask me for help with their car or their motorcycle.

I hand them candles and I tell them, in my car, I have an altar. I have my quartz, I have a dream catcher and a feather, those are to make sure that things will go well on the road, on the journey. With the candles, make the Maya cross so it is protected in the four cosmic directions. Afterward, put the candles in a fire. The dream catchers, crystals, feathers, they filter out negative energies. The sacred stones have power.

These little tips are useful. These are real ones, these little cere-monies, these practices. They are very helpful.

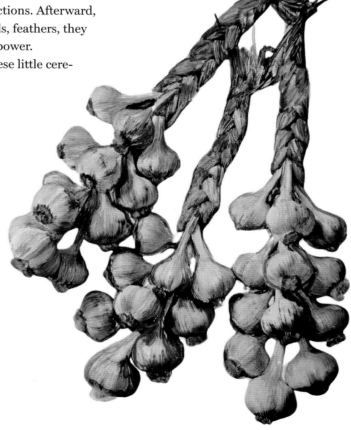

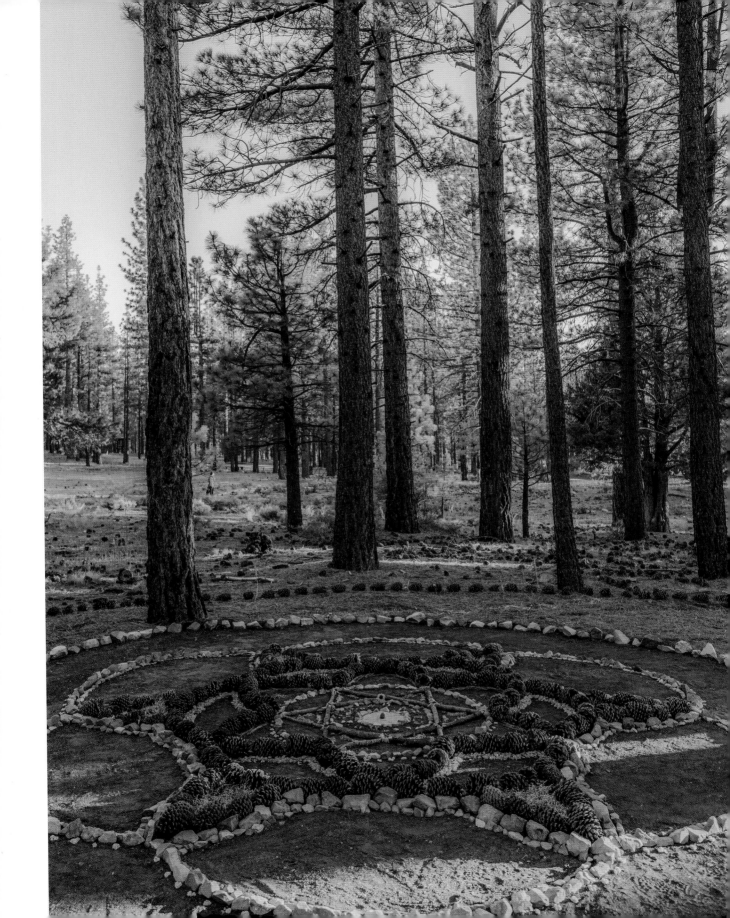

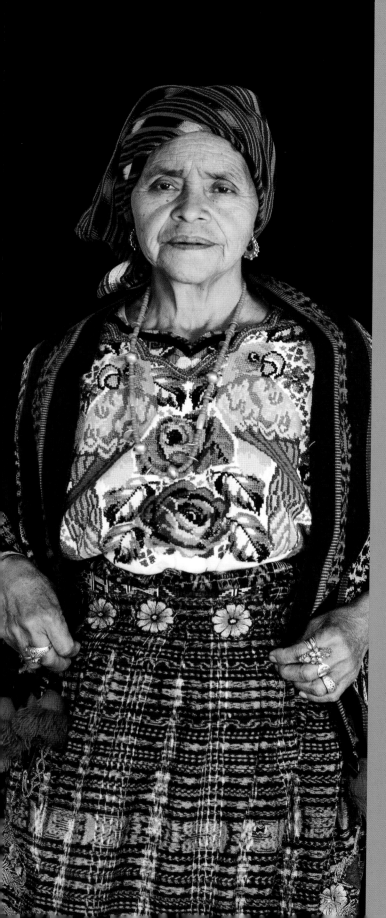

NANA ROSALÍA

Maya K'iche ✱ Guatemala

Nana Rosalía is a highly gifted spiritual guide, healer, and midwife who facilitated more than two thousand natural and conscious births without a single death or injury. With her profound knowledge, she believes a Cesarean section is never necessary, skillfully delivering babies in any position or size. Her intuitive touch allows her to determine the baby's sex simply by feeling the mother's belly.

She offers a range of holistic healing services, including abdominal massages, traditional wrapping, and heals using the sacred tobacco, Temazcal, plants, and steam baths. Her healing practices are deeply connected to the lunar cycles, ensuring alignment with natural rhythms.

Elected as part of the ancestral authorities, Nana Rosalía plays a crucial role in maintaining community order in Sololá.

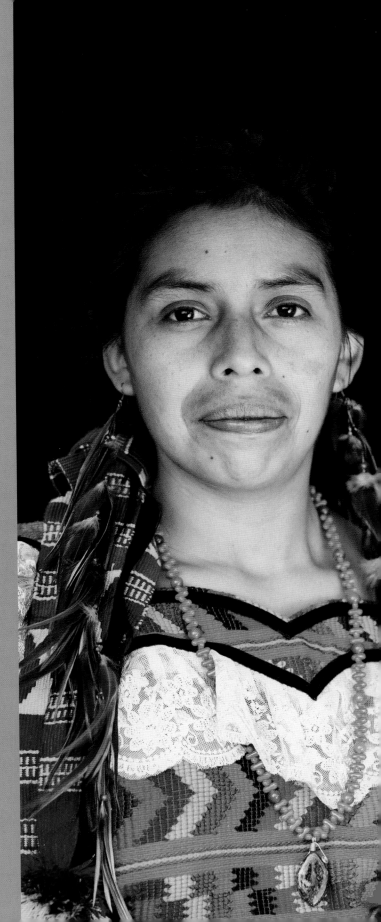

IXQUIK ZAVALA

Maya K'iche * Guatemala

Ixquik Zavala is a traditional Maya holistic midwife and a Timekeeper (Ajq'ij or spiritual guide) who works with the natural medicines of her people. As a member of the National Council of Ajq'ijab' Maya Spiritual Guides of Guatemala, she is deeply involved in the preservation and practice of her ancestral heritage.

Ixquik is a mid-level education teacher and a holistic healer midwife. She brings the ancestral wisdom, teachings, and practices of cacao medicine from the Maya cosmovision, offering profound insights and healing methods.

She is also knowledgeable about plants and skilled in Maya abdominal massage. An artisan at heart, Ixquik weaves sacred textiles on a backstrap loom, creating intricate pieces that embody cultural significance. Additionally, she conducts cosmogonic studies with Tz'ite beans (measure of time), providing spiritual guidance through this ancient practice.

Fire
Tobacco and Candles

✳

Fire is the essence of purification. Flame burns, smoke carries, and light brings. Hear from the elders about how they use the allies of fire and flame to remove energies and to call in the sacred with balance and intention.

Notice what and how the elders speak about fire through tobacco and candles.

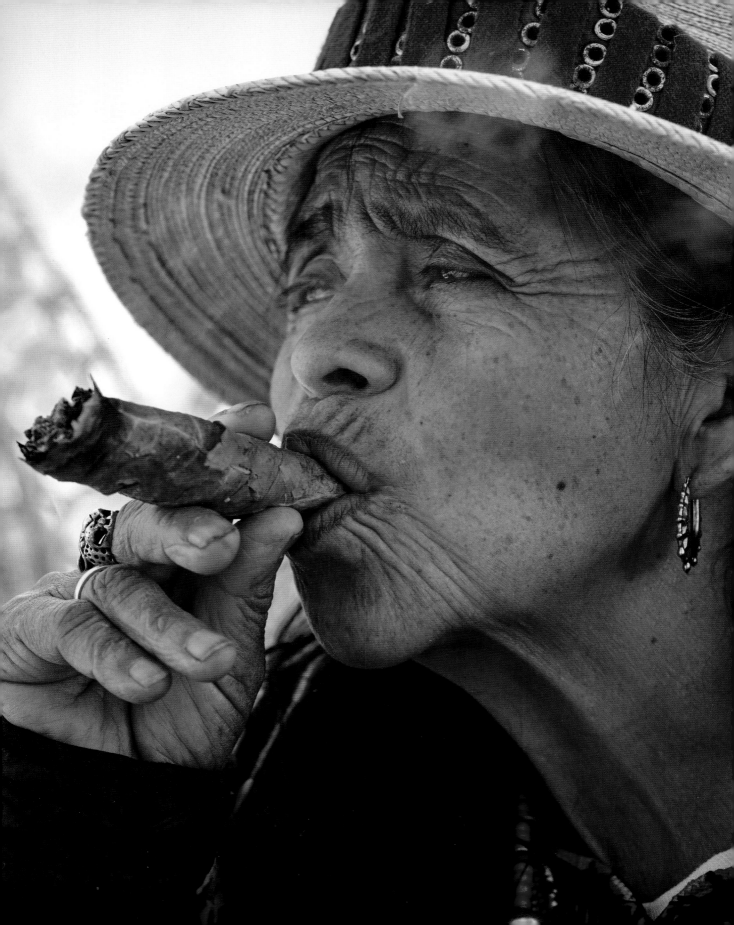

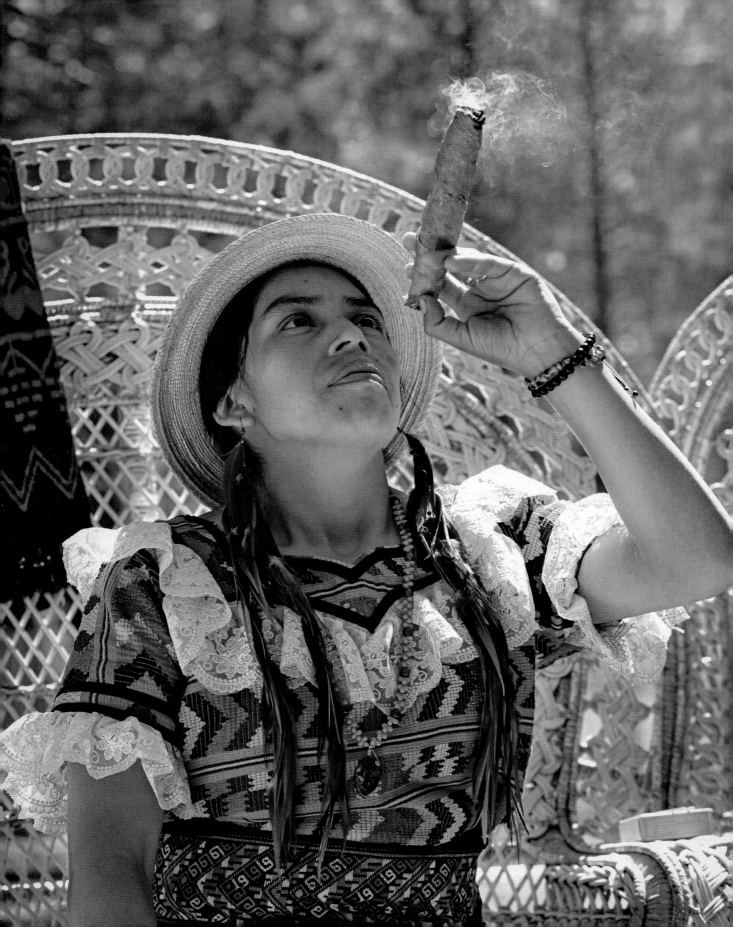

Connection with Tobacco

Nana Rosalía Zavala and Ixquik Zavala
Maya K'iche ✳ Guatemala

Tobacco is an element we find all over the world.

It is one of our main ways of connection.

We always point the tobacco upward toward the sky, to ask our ancestors for guidance; they communicate through the flame in the tobacco. The sacred tobacco is the connection.

With tobacco, we do a ceremony for people in need of freeing. It's a way to change your life. Sometimes, people say, "I feel like I can't do anything else anymore." Of course, with God, with the ancestors, there is a solution for everything in life. That's why we have the sacred tobacco.

We don't inhale the smoke into our lungs. It's just the connection, inhaling little by little but only bringing the smoke into the mouth. Three times. We raise the tobacco upward. Smoke is the connection to the cosmos. It is a personal connection honoring our present life. When we place it in the energy of the Earth's soil, we are aware of the entire creation of Mother Earth—from the smallest animals and what can be observed in the plants and elements of Mother Earth.

We also use tobacco at sunrise. We locate the four directions of fire, earth, water, and air. We locate ourselves. We make offerings to these four directions using tobacco.

We also use tobacco to cleanse our space and invoke the true presence of the Great Spirit of Creation.

It is this connection and the presence of the Great Spirit that take us to the dimensions of life.

Tobacco has a great role in our lives. It is our lifeline, our timeline that determines what we can improve, what we need to let go of, and what can come in the future.

Our tobacco has no alterations. It does not have nicotine or any other element added to it. It is pure tobacco of the Earth that grows naturally, is harvested, rolled, and dried. At the same time, we always look for a complement to the duality of tobacco—an herb to be put inside. It's like the masculine and feminine energy, but they are herbs, they are plants.

Thank you to the Maya ancestors. All the ancestors who are present through this sacred tobacco and all teachings the ancestors left us. Everything they have shared for the good of humanity.

Releasing with Tobacco

Nana Amalia Tum Xinico
Maya Kaqchiquel ✳ Guatemala

A tool that I always use in the healing I do is sacred tobacco.

Sometimes you smoke sacred tobacco, but for me generally, it is just talking to tobacco. It's talking. Through this important element that comes from the Earth, you can purify your life. Speaking, doing your prayer, asking for everything you need, all your healing, done through tobacco, which is a medicinal plant that projects us toward liberation and feeds our spirit.

Tobacco is so important that when you use it for prayers, everything is cleansed. Many times, I knead the tobacco with a little alcohol, which can be massaged for joint pain, headaches, foot massages. Kneading that tobacco just with a little liquor, then handling it with faith. Its medicinal use has its spiritual energy—it heals and cleanses like it cleanses space.

I sometimes also recommend it to people when they say their house is very cold, or they hear noises, or their furniture moves. I tell them to take some charcoal, and, whether with an incense burner or a frying pan, light it on fire. Find your little tobacco and put it in the coals and saturate your entire house with the smoke—in all your corners, on your furniture, in your bedroom, on your pillow. Especially people who suffer from insomnia, who say it is difficult for them to sleep, I tell them to do this to cleanse throughout their space. It's important to cleanse the space so there is harmony. Through tobacco, we can do that clearing. Both as a human being and for the space where we live.

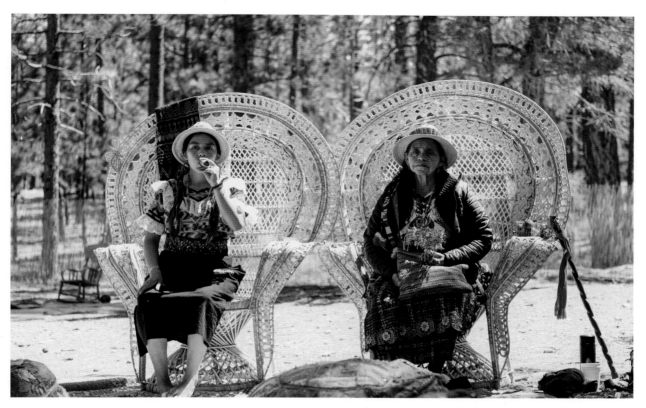

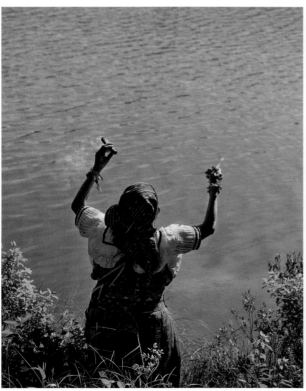

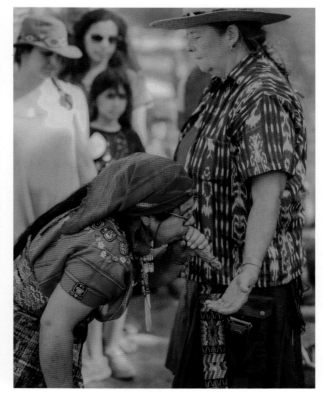

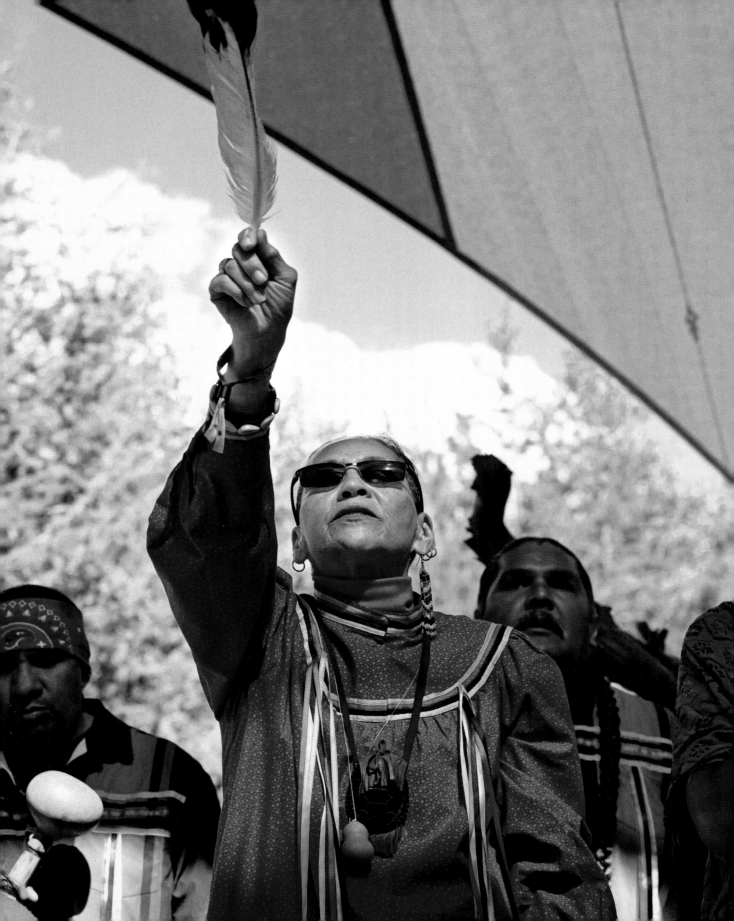

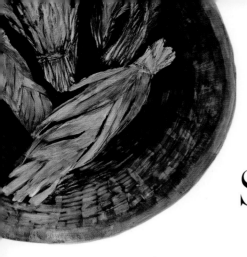

Smudging Before You Enter

Grandmother Clara Soaring Hawk
Ramapough Lenape ✳ United States

I always carry tobacco. Always.

It's so important to bring tobacco and to state your intention before you enter any new lands. To speak why you've come and carry your intention deep within your heart. You must know why you are headed to a place. I don't just show up anywhere. I feel pulled, called to bring something, to give the land something. Whatever it is I'm going there for, I make that very clear.

I greet the guardian. I greet the natural elements. Always bring tobacco. State your intention. Say why you came, knowing your heart before you get there. Why? I will give a brief explanation of what the tobacco represents and why you bring it.

Tobacco, in our nation's beliefs, is the first of the four medicines planted (tobacco, sage, cedar, sweetgrass). The roots go deep into Mother Earth and the leaves grow high. We use tobacco for prayer. You can place it in a pipe for prayer. We don't inhale tobacco because it's not to be inhaled. Your prayer is received through the burning of the tobacco. The smoke carries your prayers up. You can also release the tobacco to a spot on the ground. When you pray, hold the tobacco in your hand and, afterward, place it on the ground and know your prayers are still received. They're being drawn in through Mother Earth.

Another thing I do is smudge myself. I use sage to clear the air, to make sure that I am clear of any bad energies. The sage will pull it. We'll put it under our feet, around our head, pull it to our face, our heart. That clears any negative energies, so you don't bring any attachments.

Sage is also one of the four medicines given to us. It is to purify the air. It cleans the air. It rids, it chases away negative energy, bad energy, bad spirits. That's why you see many people using sage wands doing ceremonies clearing rooms of negative energy. Wherever you burn the sage, the negative energy disappears. The smoke from sage will clear all negative energy.

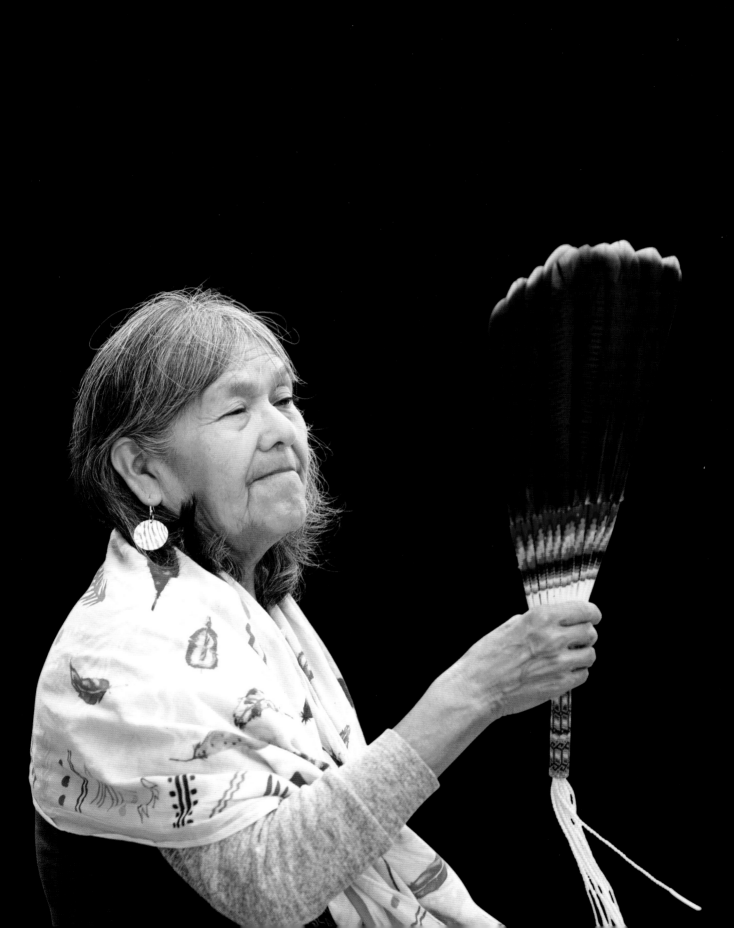

Finding Balance When the Whole World Is Shaking

Grandmother Mona Polacca
Hopi, Havasupai, Tewa ❊ United States

*How do we find balance
when the whole world is shaking?*

When there's such chaos occurring in the world, how do we find our sense of balance to hold on to the beauty of life and not get overwhelmed by what we see of man's inhumanity to man. When I say "man," I mean men and women, all of life, children, the unborn—the inhumanity and the way of destruction and chaos we're seeing. How do we come to a place where we find our sense of well-being?

I was told by my mother that there's always a time when we feel a sense of loss, we feel there's no sense of direction. There's a sense of not knowing what to do, like this place is not safe. She told me, everyone has a time in their life when they go through these things. This is part of life's challenges. Our response to the challenges is to pay attention. She said what you do is you just find a quiet spot.

Find a place where you could build a little fire in front of you. Sit in front of it and have a container of water with you. Have a plant, some plant life. It doesn't have to be a giant bush, even just one little leaf or just one little sprig of a plant. Have it there with you.

Sit down and be with those things that are of divine creation. They are not man-made. They are of a power that is beyond us. Look into that fire. Sit with the water. That water represents clarity—clarity that you're seeking in your mind, heart, body, and spirit. Sit there with it. Meditate and seek guidance.

How you seek guidance is to acknowledge, "I am in need of guidance. I need help. I don't know what to do. I feel lost. I feel sad. I feel like I don't know what to do." To acknowledge this, about how you're coming to this, is to humble yourself to it. You humble yourself to the Creator and all the spirits. Acknowledge and ask for help.

You can even cry. That's being humble. We say sometimes, "We have to go back." Sometimes, we have to go back to the basic things in life. Those are the basic things in life that you're sitting there with. So, you humble yourself. Get down on your knees. You're on Mother Earth in one of the humblest ways: on your knees or sitting and humbly shedding tears, humbly opening your heart. Humbly acknowledge the thoughts you have. You know your feelings. All of them, without holding anything back.

You release. Go ahead. Turn it over to those things that are of a great creation. They are not man-made. Go ahead and bear your heart in the humblest way.

When you're through doing that, reach out toward that fire and rub your hands together like you're washing them, then bring them to touch your heart. Put that warmth, that love, that compassion, that light that the fire represents into your heart. Touch your mind to put that light and that warmth and that compassion in your mind. Go ahead and pat your knees and your body. Bless yourself with it.

Do the same with the water. Bless yourself. Put your fingers into the water and then rub your hands together like you're washing them. Touch your heart again and your mind, and touch your feet, your knees, and bless yourself with the water.

Then, pick up that plant, that little leaf or sprig or branch. It's always good to smell it. Whatever it is. Smell the aroma of that plant because it's something of beauty. That way, you're receiving the beauty of that plant life as well. Pick it up, dip it in the water. Then, brush yourself with it, blessing yourself with it. Bless your heart. Bless your mind. Bless your body. Bless your hands and bless yourself with it.

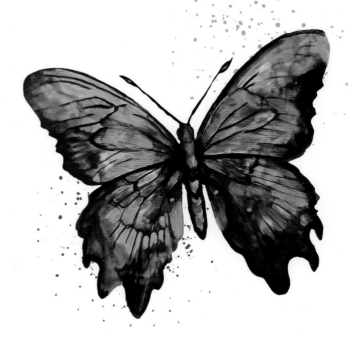

You can bring yourself back in balance. If you're outside already, or if you're inside, go out, and stand facing the direction of the sun. Face it. Reach up to it. Rub your hands together again. Touch your heart and touch your mind. Reach down to the Earth. Touch the Earth. Touch your toes and your knees and your heart and your mind again. Bless yourself. You are blessing yourself out there.

Then, what I do is reach back out to the sun. Take some of that light from the sun and put it on my face like I'm washing my face with it. Then, put some on my heart. I put my arms around myself and give myself a big hug.

When I do that, I feel so rejuvenated and happy because I feel that sense of love that comes from these creations. It's back to the basics. You've gone back to those basic things that give you life. You can be energized by it. Feel the energy of this creation that gives us every bit of life no other person gives you.

You know you have that power. Of course, our mothers know because they bear us, they carried us. Outside in this world we live in, that we grow in, there isn't any other person who gives you life. We have to maintain our life through our connection with these divine creations.

These are good practices. For me, anyway. I do that with my children. Now, I do it with my great-grandchildren. I bless them every day. Even if they're not with me, I send my blessing each and every day to them. I tell them, "I may not be there with you, but believe me, the moment I wake up, I think of you and I send you good blessings. I pray for wherever you look that daylight comes your way. Know that Grandma's love is there with you." That's what I tell them.

In that way, we can extend the blessing beyond ourselves. This is what I was told. It's in sharing it that you keep it. In that way, I share this with you and you can share it. It's not mine. I don't own it.

I give you blessings that way.

Maya Cross for Life

Tata Mario Simón Ovalle Chávez
Maya K'iche ∗ Guatemala

Candles in a cross that represents your life.

The red, top, candle is the direction of the ancestors. It represents strength. It is the red corn, red beans: elements of life.

The white, center, candle is the Nahual, the energy, of your birth. This is like the sunrise. It represents clarity in all one's actions. Purity. It is the white corn, white beans, the white flowers.

The black, bottom, candle is your destiny. This is like the sunset. It represents the messages that occur in dreams. It is the black corn, the black beans.

The yellow candle on the left and the blue and green candles on the right are for balance. The yellow represents the water that runs through our veins, our body. It is the yellow corn, the chickpeas, the flowers. It is sacred for healing. The green represents hope, vegetation, everything natural that is green. It is our hands and how we use them. Blue represents the infinite space our voice reaches through prayer. Rivers are blue because they have no end. These are the infinite life after death. We are matter, but we are also spirits.

When you do this ceremony, you thank the ancestors for taking care of your path, for taking care of your family. To the heart of sky, heart of the Earth, the ancestors say, "Thank you for my life. Thank you for what I am today and what I did today."

It is a ceremony to bring harmony.

If you had difficulties, perhaps it was for learning. If everything went perfectly, show appreciation.

One has to express oneself. One has to express both the gratitude and the needs they have. This is how you start the day and end the day.

If you travel and don't have candles, maybe carry some stones? Use stones instead of candles and talk to them and say all your prayers. Or put flowers, or food. Show that gratitude for what you have. Take 5 to 10 minutes to do this.

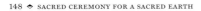

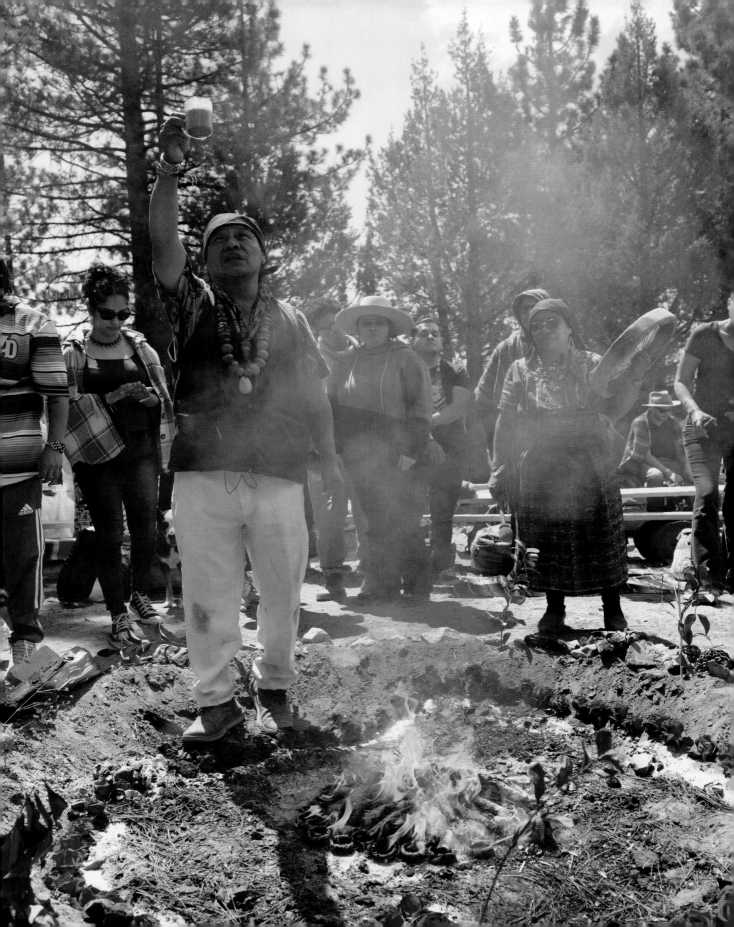

TATA MARIO SIMÓN OVALLE CHÁVEZ

Maya K'iche ⁑ Guatemala

Tata Mario is a renowned spiritual leader, naturopath, painter, and talented traditional musician. He plays the marimba, drums, caracol, and flute.

Founder of the council of Ajq'ijab' (spiritual guides) Iq B'alam and Accessor of Indigenous Townhall of Santa Lucia, Utatlán, Sololá, he gives conferences about medicinal plants, Maya cosmology and history, and advocates for the rights of Indigenous People. He's also a primary school teacher.

Tata Mario works alongside his wife, Nana Amalia, on healing, purification, and spiritual balancing ceremonies and Maya astrology readings, among other traditional ceremonies.

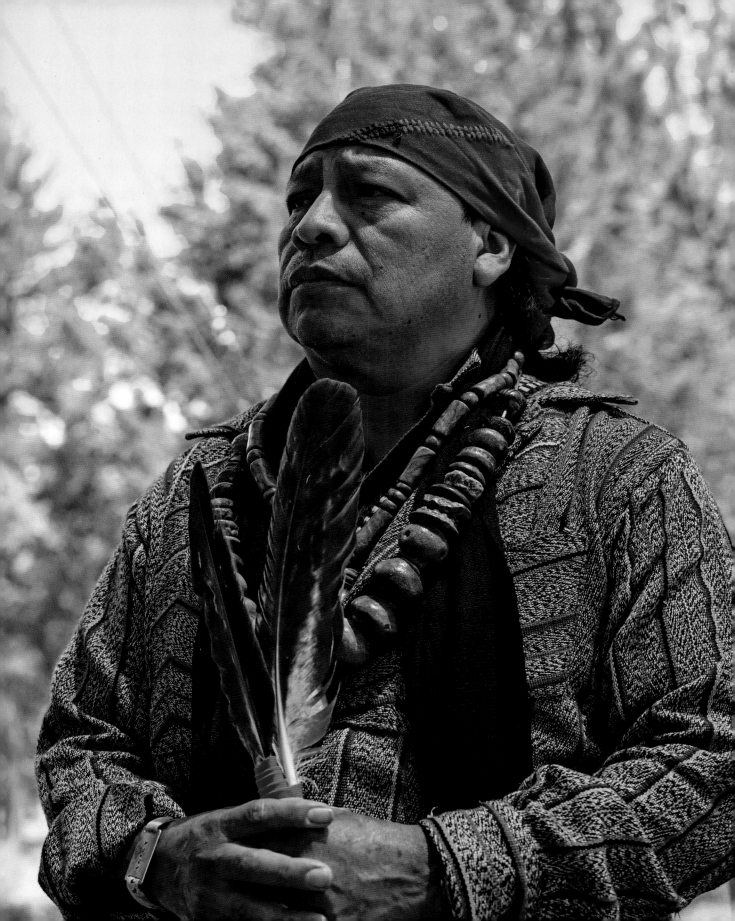

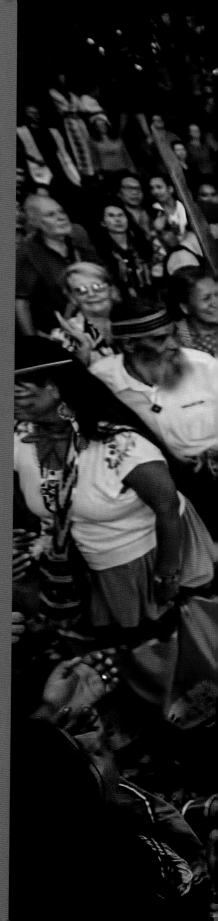

Conception
Manifesting and Creating

✳

Conception is the act of creation. From the first spark of an idea to the very act of birthing life, to be human is to participate in a multitude of acts in service to creation. Hear from our elders about how they approach the creative process as well as identity through everyday acts and deeply intentional ceremonies.

——————

Notice what and how the elders speak about conception through manifesting and creating.

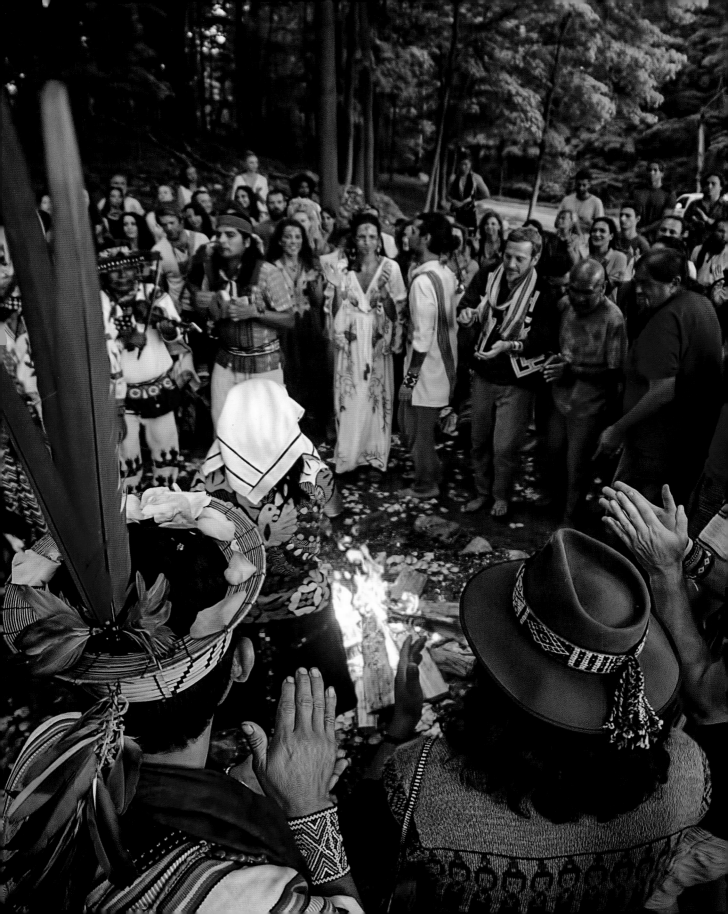

Awakening Your Creator

Louis Te Kouorehua Kereopa (Matua)
Māori ✳ New Zealand

I do not know who you are, but I would like to get to know you.

I heard that you are a creator.

I heard that you are a divine being.

I would like to have a personal relationship with you.

I know in my heart and believe in myself that you and I are not separate.

We are one and the same because we are love.

Words like this, in their simplicity, can be shared as a prayer.

The Creator wants to hear your voice. Not some voice coming out of a book or some other person who's been doing prayers for however long. Just express yourself from the heart, that's what keeps it fresh and meaningful.

Every day say, "Good morning, my friend. Thank you for the sun. Wow. It's amazing, you know?" Just a conversation. It's not being crazy. It's just you talking to your guardians, your higher self. You're talking to Creator.

The live stream of the Creator flows through us continuously. This is why we are alive. That's why we are here. It's continuous. That's his gift to us. It's why he created; it just flows through our whole being. It is never ending. It never stops. There's no judgment in that because love is love is love is love. It doesn't know anything else. Only love.

Prayer is about talking.

Practices for Conscious Conception

Nana Rosalía Zavala and Ixquik Zavala
Maya K'iche ❖ Guatemala

If one wants to have a baby, there are some plants we use to make creams and ointments that are applied to warm the uterus.

You can also take a bath with plants so the energies are strong. There are women who have a very cold body, so they massage themselves with plant creams to activate the energies in their body.

We make the creams with fresh plants. The seven plants we use are apasote, basil, chamomile, cypress, eucalyptus, pericón, and rosemary. We look for odd numbers. An odd number is like the person, the faith, the trust. If you find four kinds of plants, then to balance find a fifth. Or, you can search for all seven. The more plants you put in the preparation, the stronger it will be.

For the cream's base, use beeswax with olive oil. Put everything in a pot and place it on the fire. Bring the fresh plants with olive oil and beeswax to a boil. The plants' properties absorb into the beeswax and oil in 8 to 10 minutes. Then, strain into a jar and store.

You can also take baths or steam your genitals with these same plants.

Massage is also used. Abdominal massage, because for both the man and for the woman, the energy of the genitals is activated to conceive. Couples can do it together. The man massages his partner and the woman massages her partner.

The best time to activate these abdominal massage energies is with the lunar effects of the waning quarter, waxing quarter, new moon, or full moon. With this massage, we cleanse the contraceptives that have been in place, which have had an effect on both bodies. We have to clear these medications that also damage the human body and sometimes cause problems conceiving. The massage helps release.

Do this 7 times, minimum.

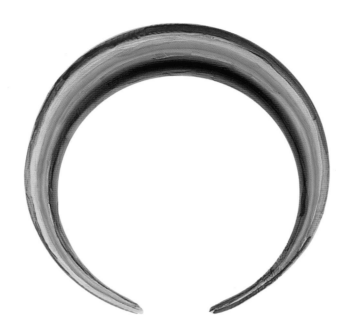

Building a Relationship with the Rainbow

Grandmother LánéSaán Moonwalker
Yoeme and Apache ❋ United States

From my heart of hearts to all of yours, I send my greetings and my love and gratitude for your beingness.

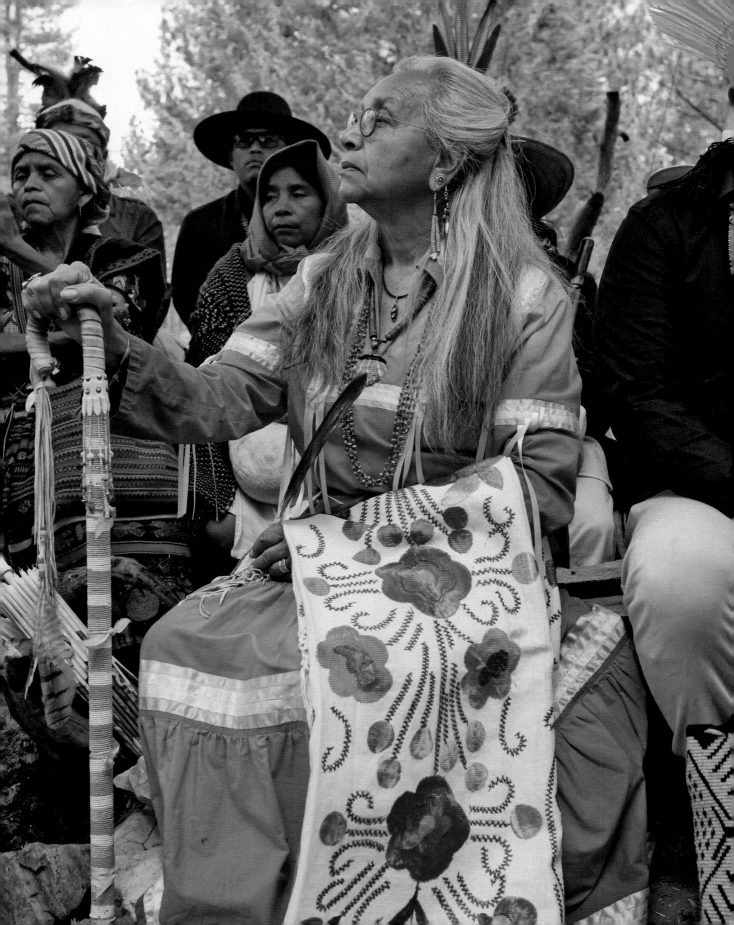

Today, we are going to share and explore how one builds a relationship with the rainbow. The reason I am willing to share this is because the rainbow from all around the world is an extremely important, sacred alliance—and always has been.

From the Abrahamic Peoples, the rainbow represents the promise from the sacred divine for peace. If you are Abrahamic in your lineage, you will remember the story of Noah. After the rains stopped, a rainbow went from one side of the horizon to the other. There was also a dove carrying an olive branch for peace. Noah was given a message at that time that there would not be water the next time, but fire instead. I hope you register that we are in those times now.

There are wars and genocides all over the world. It is a more important time for us who are following a sacred path to work with the rainbow and its promise. For Native Peoples from the Americas, we perceive the rainbow as a beingness.

Yes, we work with it as a symbol, but it is more. You will see it often in our artwork, in our iconography. This is how we work with it. Many people from other parts of the world, such as Oceania and Africa, also understand that the rainbow is a beingness. It is an elemental that has wisdom, knowledge, presence, and life. For those of us who are of the desert peoples of Turtle Island, the rainbow is a bridge of communication. It represents the journey between the sacred spirit realm and we who are physical. All of our angels, deities, and guardian spirits that guide us communicate with us through the rainbow bridge.

As a young person, I often heard, "Put your prayers forward through the rainbow bridge. Ask that your prayers be carried to the sacred spirit realm where your ancestors reside."

We have two major windows: our eyes. We also have a major window in our heart of hearts. When I say, "heart of hearts," it is not just the physical heart that is actually over on the left, but it is our whole heart center. This is the place inside us where Divine-Sacred-Energies-That-Move-All connect with us. Here, all the spirit beings, including the rainbow, lead and guide us through the rainbow bridge.

We consider the butterflies, birds, and flowers to be guardians of the rainbow, for they carry it in their beingness. All their colors is how they do this. For us, these alliances are the breathing representatives of the rainbow.

Understand that part of the bridge is already built inside you; all of us are indigenous to Hom Eh. This is a natural part of being her children. We forget this in the modern world of distraction.

We need every single color in our life, and that is why we are designed with eyes that have the ability to perceive all the colors of the rainbow. Even people who are "color blind" have some ability to discern different colors and shades.

A place to start is to make gifts and offerings to the representatives that are closer, such as the butterflies. How do you do that? Well, that's pretty easy in today's world. You buy these fancy feeders at the garden shop so we are butterfly recruiters. Traditionally, we plant flowers as well as vegetables in our gardens. You can provide a space for the flowers and the pollinators in a pot on a patio or balcony. This exchange will help you get back into the cycle of life.

If you listen to our language, we describe an ongoing exchange of energy. We're describing relationships. It is a circle of life. It is the movement between Sun Father, Earth Mother, and Grandmother Moon. We are simply a part of this. So, when you are gardening, you are engaging with this circle. Do this in a sacred way. Praying and singing is a good way to engage.

It is better for you to create the song. Our creativity is one of the few ways we humans have to give honestly. I give my plants in the garden cornmeal and tobacco. In truth, the cornmeal and tobacco are not actually mine. They are on loan from the plants who are also children of Earth Mother. My song, my breath, and my creativity are what I am truly giving from my heart of hearts.

I recommend engaging with the rainbow in a garden or in Earth Mother's garden of wildflowers. Do not come empty handed. Make offerings and gifts. If you're a little uncomfortable singing, then share through poetry, but do your best to create that poetry yourself.

Bring water if it is a dry season. If it's your garden, you have to share water. Invite all that you love in the natural world into your heart of hearts. Give back your love and gratitude through your poetry or song.

I invite you to be spontaneous in this. This enables you to truly come from your heart center. You can describe what you're doing. "I am here giving tender care to this little miracle, to this little daisy. I am here loving these geraniums and roses." We have sunflowers where I live, found throughout the deserts and the borderlands. They are wild. I have invited them into my gardens and around my home. I take water to them and I sing to them. I thank them for feeding the finches and sparrows as well as the bees and butterflies. This is how I get into the flow of the circle of life.

As you begin to work with the different parts of the rainbow, be creative. Do some drawing, beadwork, or sewing involving the colors. With each color you work with, allow that color vibration inside of you. Do this while you are cooking, even if it is a cup of tea. Understand you are engaging with the vibration of the plant as a plant as well as its color. So, when you have an orange, understand it's not just an orange. Don't go unconscious. Engage and invite the color in. Share of its beingness with you. All food has color. Water is a color too. If you look at it in the sunlight or strong moonlight, it amplifies and reflects every color around it. When in the presence of nature, invite all of its beingness, and the rainbow it holds, within. Then, give back your love and gratitude. Do this consciously.

Work with all the colors because that's how we were designed for our best life. Our healthiest, most balanced life is when we share with all the colors of the rainbow. When you are presented with a rainbow in nature, give special thanks and gratitude. Burst out in song and recite a poem made of your love.

We perceive the rainbow as a bridge. We understood it as such because, when it comes down from the heavens after a rainfall, all is blessed in its presence.

Be back in touch with the wonderment of life. All of us had this as children. It is important not to lose this wonder in our life journey, for it is that bridge of the rainbow that we walk on to return back to the sacred spirit realm and to our ancestors in a good, safe way.

I sincerely hope this is of help to you. From my heart and beingness to all of yours, we are complete. We are whole. May the rainbow bless us all in this journey.

Thank you.

NANA AMALIA TUM XINICO

Maya Kaqchiquel ✳ Guatemala

Nana Amalia Tum Xinico is a talented healer, naturopath, and renowned spiritual leader and teacher. She is a member of the committee of the sacred sites of Guatemala, COLUSAG, founder of the council of elders Iq B'alam, member of the council of elders and political association of Maya women, MOLOJ.

Nana Amalia carries out her sacred mission alongside her husband, Tata Mario, in ceremonies of healing, purification, and spiritual balance, and divinations and analysis with the sacred Tzite (beans) in relation to the Maya lunar calendar, among other practices and Maya ceremonies of Guatemala.

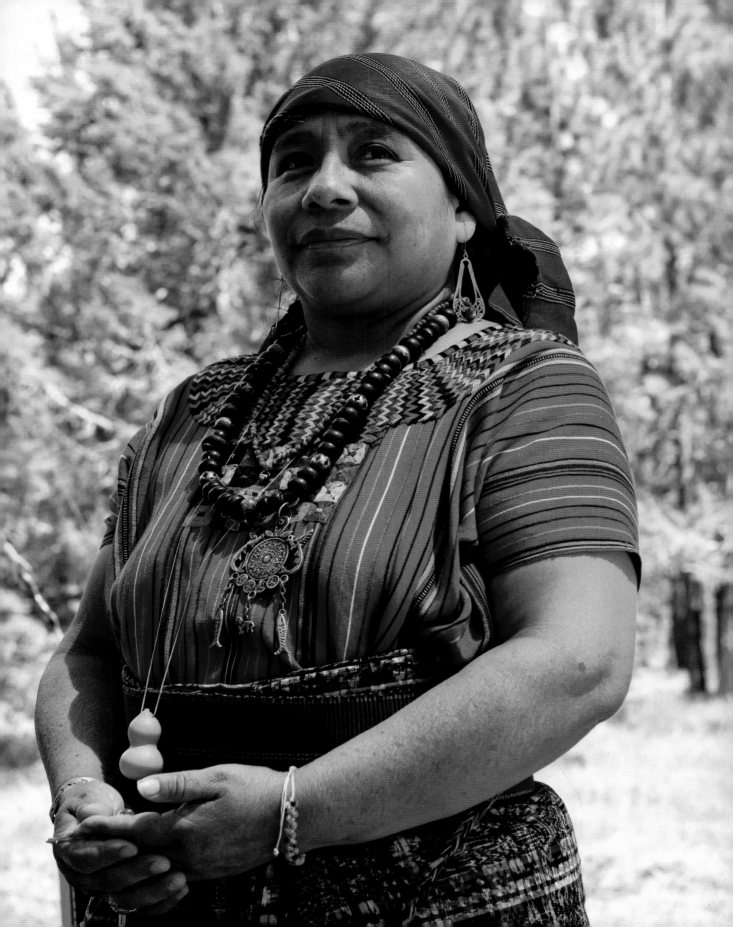

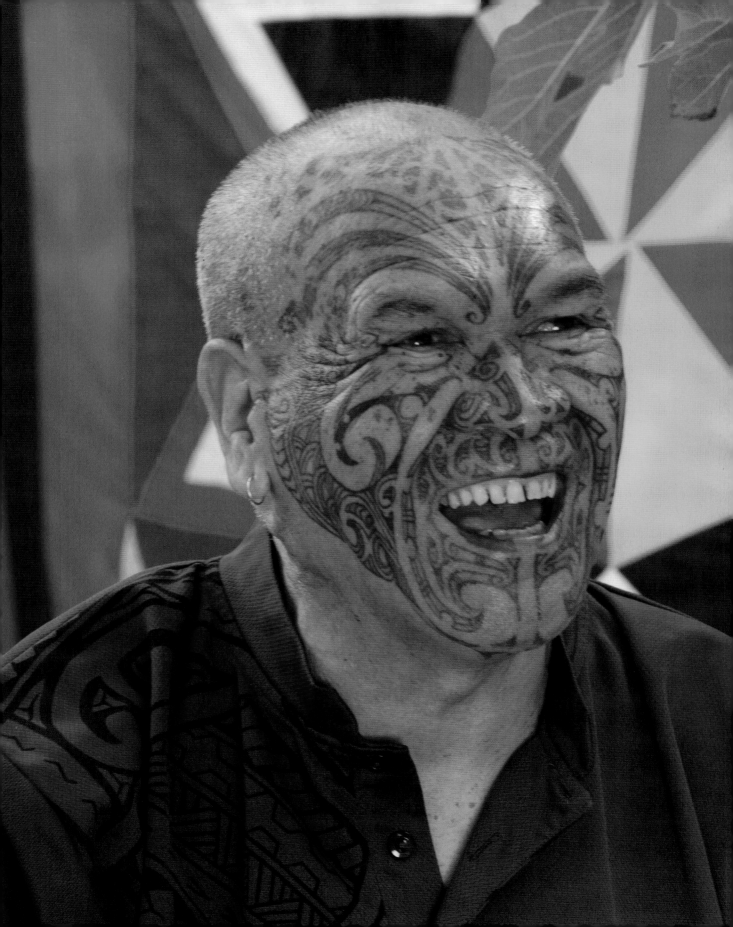

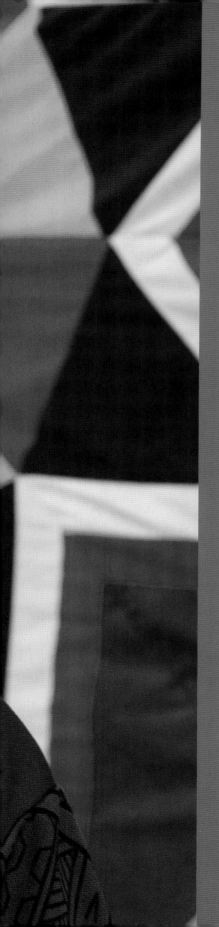

Space
Carving and Containers

✳

Space is where creation abides.
From our cosmos to our dwellings,
it is the anchoring of spirit into the
domain of our experience within both
inner and outer worlds. Hear from the
elders about how they regard the act of
making and holding space for life and
spirit to enter.

———————

*Notice what and how the elders speak about space
through carving and containers.*

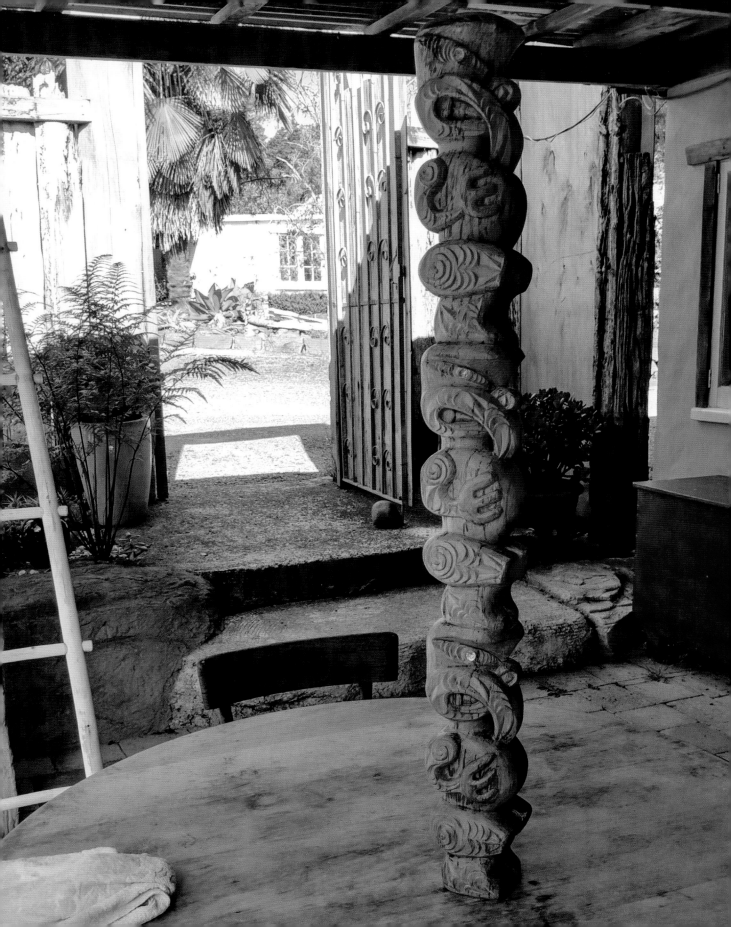

Create a Spiritual House for Your Inner Child

Louis Te Kouorehua Kereopa (Matua)
Māori ✳ New Zealand

When I grew up, I was always surrounded by carving.

Now, we call our "marae" (the sacred courtyard of a Māori meeting house, Wharepuni), our meeting place.

I'm a mystic artist. I've been given that name "mystic" by a seer. He gave that message to me, but I just work. Drawing, carving, painting, whatever form, my hands are the instruments to manifest the work.

When I do the work, it's not just me working. I know I'm surrounded by and looked after by other ancestors or other angelic beings or whoever comes in to help make the story beautiful for other people to see.

It's a story in wood, not on paper. That's my being an author. I am a master carver. I do my writing in wood. I've always been able to. I explain to people, when they ask questions about the carving, that having something in carving means only a few come to see the work. You know what? Whatever the number of people, they will see the story. It creates a domino effect. My work, whether it's a mythical, mystical story or legend that's handed down, always comes back to why we are here as humans, which is a personal journey.

There are aspects in the carvings themselves. Some simplicity of the carvings make any person who sees the carving become warm straightaway. They are drawn to the carving. They may not understand what they see, but it's the feeling you get from the carving. The carving talks to you individually, not in words, but in what you feel intuitively. That's the work.

The gift came from the Creator and I'm just continuously, on our behalf, giving that back to say thank you, thank you, thank you. Each chip, each marking, everything until it's finished is like a continuous thank you on behalf of all of us.

In the olden days, with the carvers, when a student under the tutorship of a master carver did his first carving, the master would say, "I want you to take this carving to the forest and bury it." The student, "Oh, but I created that carving. It's beautiful. It should be mine." Take it to the forest and give it back to Tāne, the guardian of the forest. Give it back to Mama. That means do not become attached to your work because, in the ceremony sense, you're going to be carving many, many things. You're going to be here for service to other people. Let it go. That's your calling.

When I was a teacher, I had a few students. I said to them, when you graduate, you will choose one carving and give it to someone who's come to the graduation—could be your mother, your girlfriend, your boyfriend, or whoever. It's a way of giving back, of separating yourself. It'll clear you so you can continue the work.

Some people refer to ceremony as the beating of the drum, but I speak about the ceremony of the heart. Expressing to manifest a service you give to others as well as yourself—that's what a ceremony is. It encompasses that whole. Yes, you have in your heart giving, and you will receive.

You have a little house, a temple inside of you. You created that temple and you know what that temple is like. You can make one, you know. It can be crystals, many colors, rainbow, whatever furniture you want to put inside. You can talk to the house, you can do anything you like. You could draw it, it might be a teepee, whatever. Whatever shape you feel is comfortable for you.

The little wooden houses I make, I have people come up, and I take off the roof. Then, they have a look inside the house and what do they see? They will see nothing. It's nothing inside the house because it's about your own mind. The mind, being like a computer, will just keep going and going. It's a tool we use. What you see will help you see your journey. What do you feel you would like to see inside the house? If you see flowers, that's good because you see it in your mind. All your troubles, look at the house and send them to the house. It's a symbol for yourself.

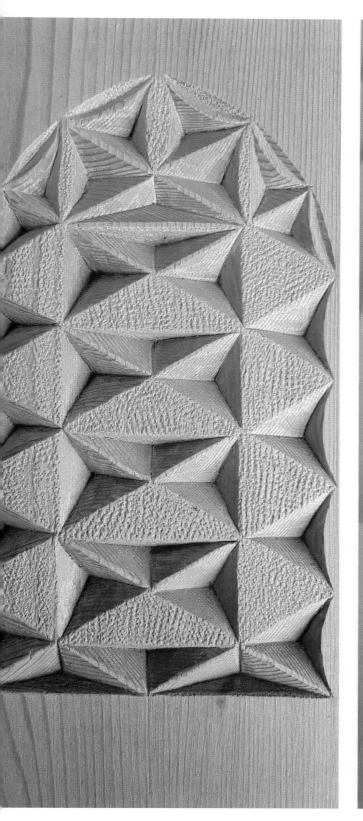
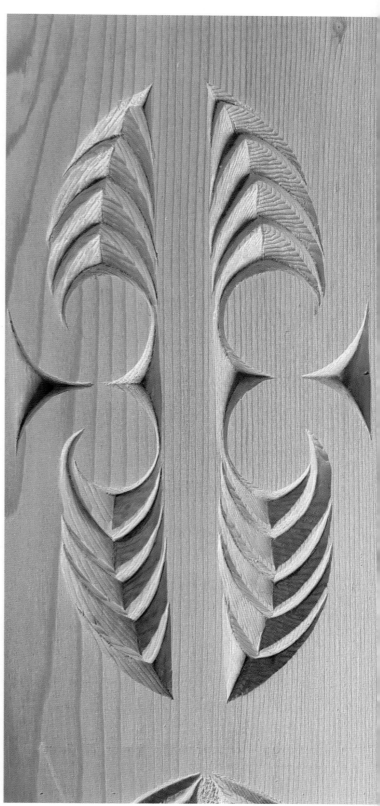

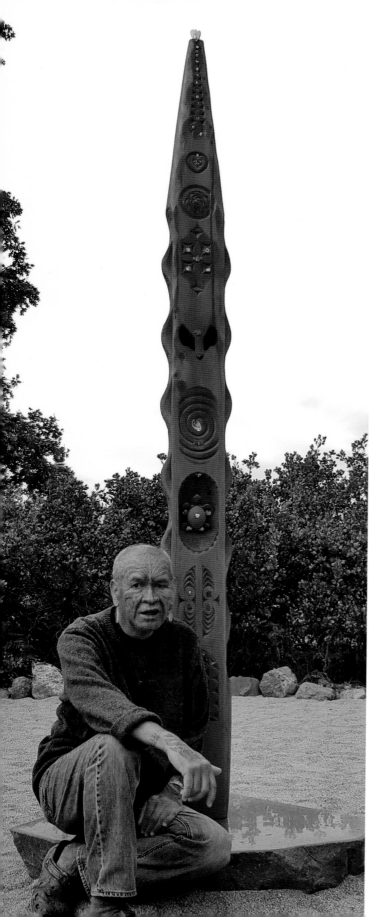
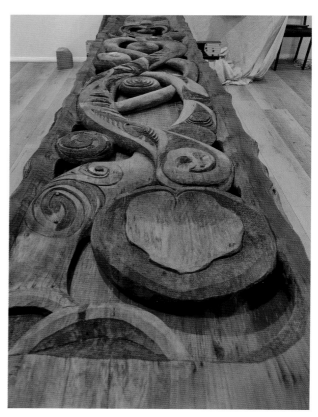
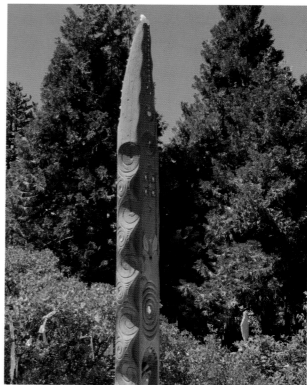

You have that little house inside of you. You know what that temple is like. That's the ceremony. In the depth of ceremony, you must always know first: Who are you?

The inner, inner, inner, of your own personal universe is what we call your "higher self." That's your inner child. It's not an energy. I helped a woman connect with her inner child and I will share. I used myself, acting it out for her to connect with my inner child. I said to my inner child, "I'm here and I've come to say I love you."

The inner child says, "No . . . no, you haven't."

I said, "Yes. I've come to see you. I've come to tell you that I love you."

"No, you don't. No, you don't. You pushed me away a long, long, long time ago. You pushed me when you were busy looking outside yourself. You forgot about me. I have been knocking on your door since I came into this world, waiting for you to greet me."

I said, "No, I've come to say I love you and I am sorry too."

"No, you haven't."

I'd keep repeating that to make myself feel warm so my inner child will feel that warmth, and then I said, "What happened a long time ago, that happened then, but I'm a grown man now. I am a grown man. I have changed. I have grown. I'm not a baby anymore. I'm not a young boy anymore. Indeed, I've learned many lessons and I'm still learning my lessons. I am sorry I had forgotten about you, but I've come today to say I love you."

"Really?"

"Yes. I love you."

"Really? You love me?"

"Yes, I love you."

Then, you have a feeling of warmth, like when a child says, "I have always loved you and will always love you." My friend, she cried when I was telling this story to her. She's fine now. Once that happens, when you wake up in the morning through the eyes of your inner child, you will see the world for the first time. And my friend, she's like a little child. Everywhere she goes, she's happy. She's had a feeling of going home to her people. She'll share the same story with those who are trying to search for something and answer for themselves.

That is a ceremonial prayer of the heart speaking to your inner soul. That inner child will keep knocking on that door until you feel that release within yourself. The house can be used like that. A little house. Oh, I've made this house! This is the house of just me and my inner child! No one else can make your own house.

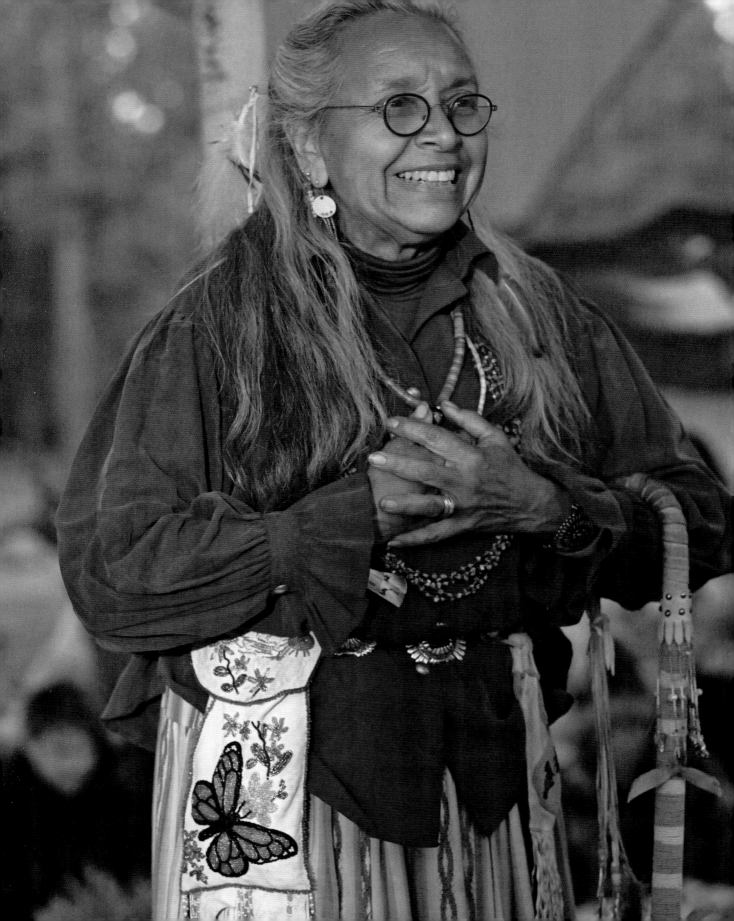

Meditating with the Full Moon

Grandmother LánéSaán Moonwalker
Yoeme and Apache ✳ United States

Greetings. I am Grandmother LánéSaán Moonwalker. As my name suggests, I have a close relationship with the moon.

I was given the name "Moonwalker" because I belong to a lineage for whom working with the moon is a daily practice. We recognize and understand that O'na He, also known as Grandmother Moon in English, is precisely that for us—our grandmother.

   She creates the gentle rocking motion that enables sentient life to exist on our most beloved Earth Mother, Hom Eh. Grandmother Moon sets our heartbeat and our breath through that rocking motion. Therefore, we consider it important to work with her on a conscious level. Whether we have a practice or not, every living being on this beloved planet is influenced by Grandmother Moon.

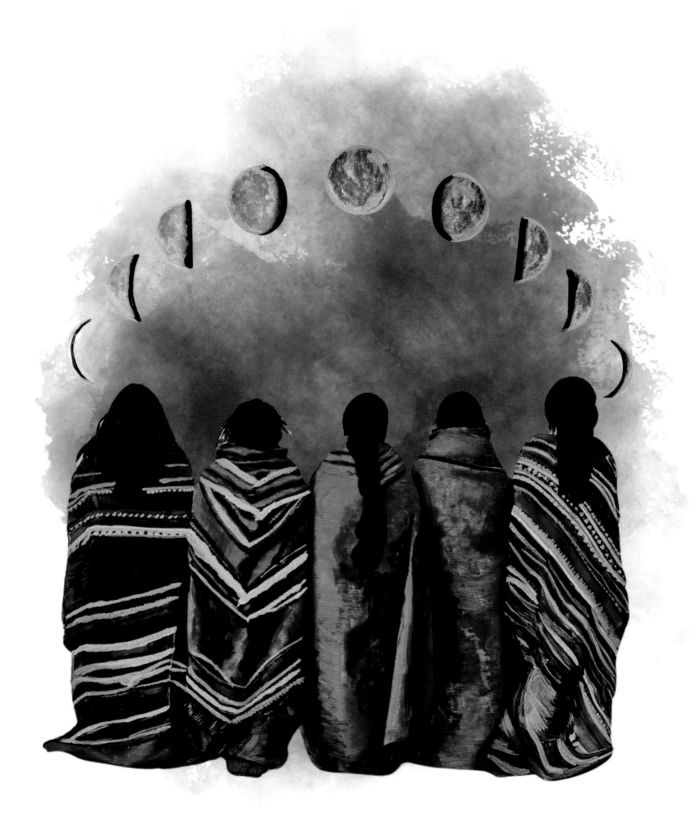

When we work with O'na He, as a way of praying, we offer song. By offering this song made of our love, we acknowledge her and the bridge of rainbow light that connects us to her. This is on all levels: physical, emotional, ethereal, spiritual, and motivational. The bridge that connects us to Grandmother Moon is the journey from the psychic and sacred spiritual realm to our physical realm. This also helps bridge internally between our psychic, spiritual, and physical self.

We consider the full moon to be the easiest time for us to connect with O'na He. We work with this part of her cycle for three nights—the waxing of the full moon, the full moon, and the waning of the full moon.

Whenever possible, we go outside to do this meditation. First, connect with Sky Father and Star Keeper above, and then Earth Mother below. To do this, we create a pool of rainbow light and energy at our heart center using the natural elements we love, rather than those created by humans. After creating this sacred energetic pool in your heart center, convert it into a beam of light.

We send our gratitude and love forth to Sky Father through this rainbow light we have created. We do this through song, and our prayers and words. Then, we send a beam of rainbow light to Earth Mother. Do your best to stay in a place of humility and love as you do this practice.

If you play a musical instrument, such as a flute, utilize it to enhance your connection with nature during this process. Once we are in as much alignment as possible, we offer a special prayer of gratitude to Grandmother Moon. We offer a sound that we are inspired to share when facing the moon, and it emanates from our voice and breath as a rainbow beam of light. Then, we ask her to reflect a rainbow beam of light from her in the sacred spirit realm to us at our heart center. Since we are engaging with the ethereal realm, it is essential to speak these words in our own way and make them personal. In this way, we make our request for Grandmother Moon to share back with us.

The purpose of this practice is to receive help in creating a bridge between the realms. Once this is done, with the help of Grandmother Moon, I promise you, you will feel it. It will be there in your heart of hearts. Some of you may feel it in your hands or a sense of expansiveness as well. This can be ungrounding. Once you are in that place of connection with her, speak of your love and gratitude for her, for your life, and for the very breath you take.

Without this connection, neither you nor I would exist. It would not exist for the trees, birds, and animals, or even the living waters. All of life is dependent on this connection to the moon and, therefore, the first and most important part of your gratitude prayers should be for this gift of life, death, and beingness.

Now, you can start the process of asking Grandmother Moon for help with clarity and a more pure heart in addressing the challenges of your life. Don't try to tackle them all at once. Take it one thing at a time. If there is something that is particularly bothering you, address that first. If you need guidance in understanding some past experiences, pick one and ask her to help you clarify and gain understanding by illuminating what is hidden and in the dark. This is her job. In addition to providing the rocking motion necessary for life, which is sentient, she also lights our way in the dark—whether it's outside of us during the nighttime or inside of us, hidden by us from ourselves. It's not a comfortable process to look at our less than beautiful or exemplary aspects. It's necessary for us to confront our fears, angers, and grief. We must address our shadows. If we do not do this, we will not be able to open our heart centers and experience love and joy in a truly good and pure way.

This is where we begin. For us of the Southwest, Yoeme and Apache, we address our inner world first. We know that our greatest enemy is inside of us. If I want to show up with clarity, authenticity, transparency, and honor in my interactions with others, I first need to work on the enemy within. Otherwise, I can think that I am telling you the truth but, in reality, it may be a lie I am telling myself. This is why we seek Grandmother Moon's help. She helps us see ourselves clearly—including our strengths and our weaknesses. She helps clarify how we perceive others, and their strengths and weaknesses. Sometimes, we may not be willing to face the truth about ourselves and our situations, and that's where Grandmother Moon comes in. She sees everything and can help us navigate through the darkest parts of ourselves to find the light.

By offering our worst and best parts to Grandmother Moon in this way, we can release that material with her radiant psychic fire, her light. This gives us the opportunity to clear away any illusions or distortions and perceive reality as it is. It's important to work with what is real, rather than a fantasy in our head. It is necessary to make meaningful changes in our lives and destiny. Only by facing and addressing our true selves can we move forward with greater clarity, authenticity, and humility.

Grandmother Moon has the capacity to perceive and understand us from a place of neutral acceptance. She is not deceived by illusions or delusions. Through the rainbow bridge (see page 158), we can invite her psychic fire into us, and we can learn to be more neutral and accepting of ourselves and others. This includes everything from our pets, the land we live on, the country we live in, our loved ones, and even our enemies. It encompasses all of life, including the final process of death.

With this song, after offering up each part of ourselves, it is important to remember to focus on one negative (weakness) and positive (strength) aspect of ourselves at a time during each meditation with Grandmother Moon. The negative side includes our fears, whether they are reasonable or not. Fear takes energy and is, therefore, a negative, not in a punitive Abra-

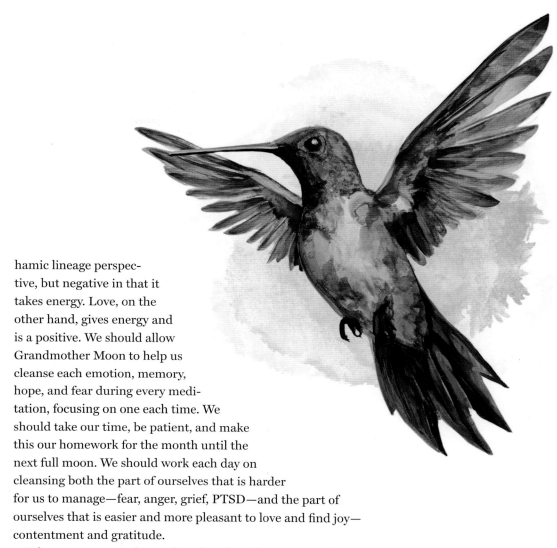

hamic lineage perspective, but negative in that it takes energy. Love, on the other hand, gives energy and is a positive. We should allow Grandmother Moon to help us cleanse each emotion, memory, hope, and fear during every meditation, focusing on one each time. We should take our time, be patient, and make this our homework for the month until the next full moon. We should work each day on cleansing both the part of ourselves that is harder for us to manage—fear, anger, grief, PTSD—and the part of ourselves that is easier and more pleasant to love and find joy—contentment and gratitude.

When you are complete, take a deep breath. Go to your heart center. Take another deep breath. Now, place there that which you love, which is natural, not human. Convert it into a pool of rainbow light and energy. And through that rainbow bridge, send back to Grandmother Moon your prayer of gratitude and love. Allow her to send back to you, through that sacred rainbow bridge, acceptance and love of you.

With that, bring closure to your meditation and prayer. Release the rainbow bridge between O'na He and you. Be creative. Be intuitive. If you are moved to do a dance of love and joy in honor of this, then do so. If you are inspired to sing or to speak a poem or pray, chant, then do that. When it is complete, take a moment to rub your hands together, warm them, and gently place them on your heart center, one hand on top of the other, with your thumbs touching each other. Know you are complete and in greater alignment with the whole.

With that, I give you my thanks and gratitude. The circle is complete and we are one with it.

GRANDMOTHER LÁNÉSAÁN MOONWALKER

Yoeme and Apache ✳ United States

LánéSaán Moonwalker has been an oracle, healer, spiritual teacher, and environmental guardian for most of her life.

LánéSaán began her training in the healing arts at the age of 12 from members of her family who were highly skilled curanderas (traditional healers who combine Native and Catholic spiritual beliefs and practices). She learned to work with creative expression as a doorway to spirit, with her mother as her first teacher.

LánéSaán is an accomplished artist, weaver, and painter as well as a dancer and singer, and she holds a degree in humanities and the visual arts from the University of Colorado. She has been a licensed minister for more than 42 years and is a Canon in the Brigade of Light.

LánéSaán has studied with many spiritual teachers, including artist, writer, and visionary Joseph Rael (Beautiful Painted Arrow), Eric Tao, and Marian Starnes.

In 1987, she met her main teacher and mentor, Tu Moonwalker, an Apache, the great-great-granddaughter of Cochise. Tu was the holder of this unbroken Moonwalker lineage. LánéSaán is an acknowledged part of that in addition to being from an unbroken lineage herself through her Yoeme grandmother. Together, Tu and LánéSaán founded the Philosophy of Universal Beingness within the Whole. The foundation of this system is about working with nature in a sacred way.

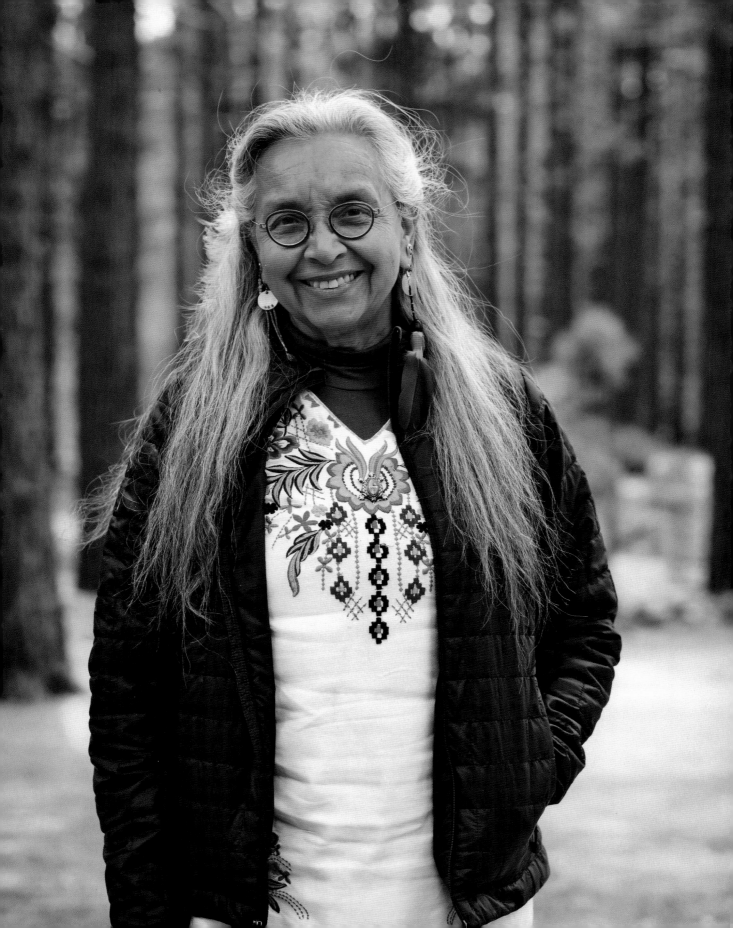

Time

Cycles and Energy

✳

Time is rhythm. It is the dance of life that gives energy to the cosmos. Hear from our elders about how they dance with the rhythms of time and synchronize the steps of life to creation's beats. Held in the embrace of time's steady ebbs, flows, and grooves are ceremonies to help us keep in alignment with our true mission and purpose in life.

Notice what and how the elders speak about time through cycles and energy.

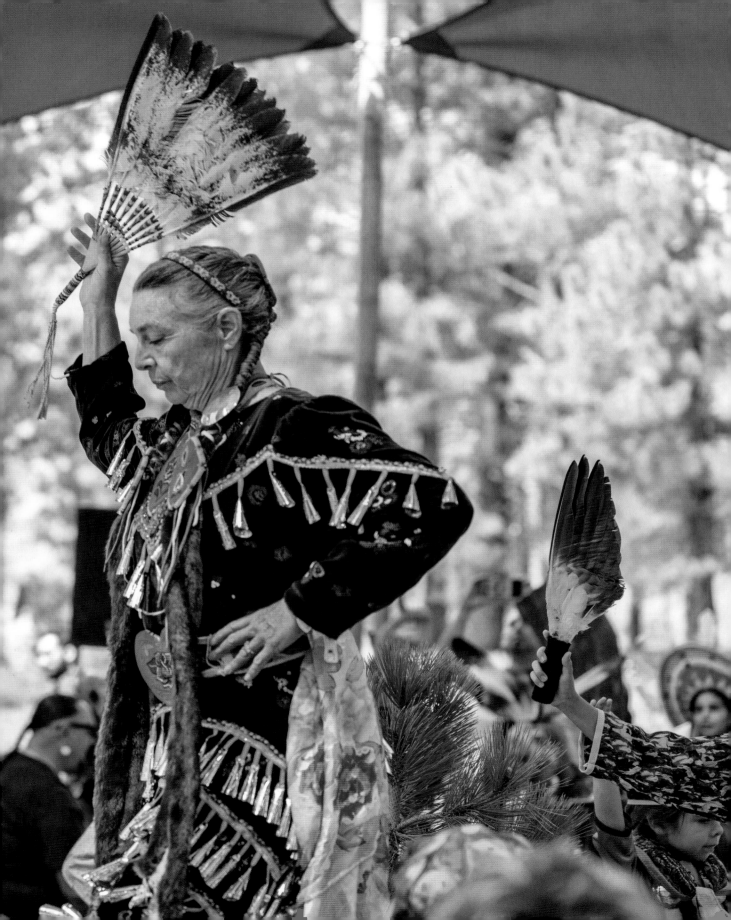

The 20 Nahuals of the Maya Lunar Calendar CHOLQ'IJ

Nana Amalia Tum Xinico
Maya Kaqchiquel ⁑ Guatemala

The lunar calendar is dedicated to the personality
and characteristics of human beings.

We use it not only for healing, but also for projects, for work, to open the way, to offer, for sowing, for harvesting. The Maya calendar is a whole that is connected with everything and, just like the human being, it has its objective. If this reaches people, then it is an instrument they can use as a map to their lives, for their growth in every sense.

The Maya calendar system is called Tzolk'in. It consists of 260 days divided into 13 periods of 20 days. This lunar calendar has been passed down from generation to generation. Today, in Guatemala, we manage two calendars: the lunar and the solar. There were many calendars, but, like all of history, colonization erased everything, burned everything. We thank the elders who remained to take care of the fire, to take care of the calendar in oral form.

This has been the struggle and it has been the experience of the ancestors who maintained these calendars for thousands of years in oral form, not written. For example, I don't use a book for reference. I know the names of the Nahuals, the energies, for each day. It's in my language. Every year in Guatemala, a brochure comes out to give us indications of what is experienced orally according to the story that appears on a stela in a sacred site called Quirigua, in northern Guatemala. It is the evidence that this calendar of ours really exists.

This calendar helps us discover our mission in life. Its 260 days are approximately the time that human gestation takes. We are talking about 13 months in the lunar calendar. We do not speak of 9 months of pregnancy; we speak of 13 months of 20 days each according to our lunar calendar. The Maya wisdom transcends the thresholds of space-time through the moon

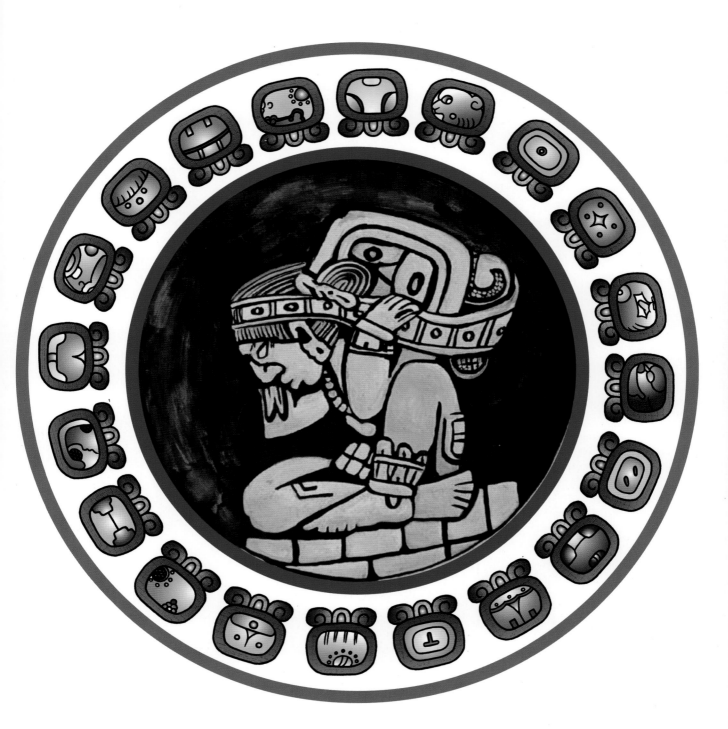

and through the stars because the lunar cycle is linked directly to this calendar. There are many accounts today about the lunar calendar; however, we, the Maya timekeepers of Guatemala, preserve and transmit this knowledge orally to new generations.

Each day of the lunar calendar has an objective. Through this calendar, a person discovers their mission. As the ancestors say, a timekeeper is not made, they are born. When they say you are "born," it means every human being brings a mission. That is why there are diverse specialties within humanity. From the Maya perspective, we are all children of a creator, Father and Mother, each person with their own strengths and weaknesses, each being is unique; therefore, we are a diversity within Mother Earth. There are artisans. There are writers. There are psychologists. There are scientists, dancers, lawyers, those who become presidents. Every healer is born with a mission. There is a diversity of human beings who have discover their mission and feel free to fulfill it. Through the lunar calendar, or sacred calendar, a person discovers their mission.

Through this calendar, we also discover our weaknesses. From birth, human beings already bring their weaknesses. Children, for example, from a very young age, already react with their weaknesses. They get a little angry; they scream; they throw a tantrum. It is because we are already born with our weaknesses, and, over time, with the growth process, the human being will search for balance and, with balance, decide what to do. What do you want to do? Do you want to bring the positive according to your Nahual? Or do you want to link yourself to the negative? So many human beings have to decide what they want to do with their life.

By discovering your mission according to the Maya lunar calendar, you could navigate each day by the different portal that opens conducive to a certain energy. In the Maya calendar, since each day has its own different energies that can be good for some people, they are like portals that open every day. Yes, each day has a specific objective. For example, in the energy of where I am today, a ceremony can be held thanking the feminine energy, thanking everything that Mother Earth gives us. We appreciate homes, whether purchased or donated. If you buy a piece of land, today is the time to open that portal and give thanks or ask to acquire material well-being. Tomorrow turns us toward the energy of harmony in which I perform ceremony or ask for business. This fits for people who have a store or are in commerce where money abounds. They have to be grateful for the job and opportunities they have. Each day in the lunar calendar gives us a specific guideline to carry out any event in our lives, whether personal, family, collective, or for humanity. There is a goal. Each day offers us an opportunity according to the lunar calendar.

The twenty Nahuals that make up the lunar Maya calendar (sacred Maya calendar) are presented here, with a brief explanation and their influence on human beings.

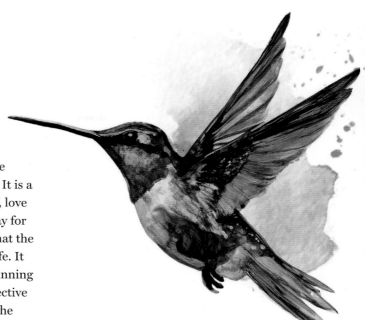

B'atz

It is recommended to consult about the destiny of a couple under B'atz energy. It is a day indicated to honor love for oneself, love for humanity, love for the couple—a day for the celebration of marriage or to ask that the compatible couple find the thread of life. It is also a time for ceremony for the beginning of any activity—personal or at the collective level. It is unity. This is the Nahual of the artist, a day to unravel marital problems so enmities do not break out and to live in harmony, in balance, with oneself and the spirit of human love and that of another being.

B'ey (or E)

This is the sacred path, a day to ask for a straight path, a clean path. Ask for a good path for travel and to undertake work, for a better future. It is also for people to clean their spiritual paths, to straighten the path of life and be guided by the Great Spirit, ask for direction and to understand what is happening around us.

Aj

Aj is the cane, the growing shoot of renewal, of family well-being. It is a day to give thanks for our children, to purify our homes with tobacco, with sacred smoke, and to give thanks for one's own life, for the mission and useful existence on Mother Earth. It is a time to ask for harmony and family well-being and to live in peace.

I'x

Symbol of Mother Earth and feminine energy, energy of the altars, ceremonial centers, it is to offer to Mother Earth for all the goodness necessary to be able to live. This is a day to pray for the animals, for domestic animals or pets, ceremony of gratitude for the land, the house acquired through time.

Tz'ikin

This represents the messenger birds, the quetzal, the eagle, the condor, the humming-bird, all the guardian birds of the forests. It is a symbol of freedom. It is to give thanks for abundance for one's work and to cleanse negative thoughts so as not to suffer poverty—spiritual and material.

Ajmaq

This gives us the opportunity to apologize, and apologize for moral forces. It is conscience, a time to mend or recognize our mistakes made and improve every day. We ask the Ajmaq and our ancestors for their intermediation so mistakes are not repeated. This is a day to heal all types of diseases and seek solutions to mental, physical, and emotional problems.

Noj

Symbol of wisdom. In this Nahual, we appreciate the knowledge acquired and transform it into wisdom. It is requested for memory and studies. The mind is freed and we ask for positive thoughts, clear thoughts.

Tijax

Symbol of the obsidian stone. For this day, a Maya ceremonial offering is made to make energy cuts for physical, emotional, and mental healing. It is a time to ask to move away from sadness, anguish, and depression. Tijax is a day of purification and balance of our actions, a day to pray for health, to prevent and free ourselves from evils and accidents.

Kawoq

Symbol of the land and the Temazcal (traditional Maya sweat lodge, considered the first hospital on Earth) Grandmother. A day to ask for the family, for the community, to ask for fertility and the good management of medicinal plants and good climate for crops. You can perform thermal baths, baths in the Temazcal (a sweat lodge in which volcanic rocks are heated and water is thrown on them, which produces steam—pure oxygen, which purifies the body, mind, emotions, and spirit) with medicinal plants, with flowers on this day.

Ajpu

Symbol of Grandfather Sun, it represents the complete being. The Grandfather Sun is asked for fire to purify our mind, which illuminates our personal, family, and collective life, and to ask for strength to overcome all types of problems or weaknesses we face as human beings.

Imox

Water, sea, brain, madness. The ceremonies of this day serve to help people with negative charges, to ask about mental problems and achieve cures, to ask to solve the different problems people face—individual or communal problems. A day to let ourselves flow like water for the cleansing and liberation of the mind from negative thinking and emotional ailments we suffer.

Iq'

Wind, air. A day for exercises for our breathing, for oxygen for our brain and vital principles. For this energy, we ask the spirit of the wind that cleanses and purifies, and ask for the healing of psychological problems, healing of passions that harm. A time for overcoming hatred and depression.

Aq'abal

A new dawn, the duality of day and night. Renewal of the stages of life. We ask for clarity for our personal, family, and collective life. We ask that we are not invaded by crying, slander, and lies, and that days of peace may dawn. May hidden things be discovered and our sacred fire and our bright inner light not go out.

Kat

Symbol of the energy and strength and heat that exists in our heart. It is the network, unity, the web of life that unites and helps free ourselves from oppression, of tangled lies or knots that do not allow us to move forward with our life. A symbol of fire, the sacred legacy of our ancestors to help us remove bad energies.

Kan

This represents the feathered serpent, which has its base in the spinal column. It is the cycle of time, authority, justice, truth. This day, the feminine and masculine are honored. It is the Nahual of sexuality, when the sacred menstruation can be offered. It is requested that there be respect and that the sexual act is sacred and in fullness. Another request is made for the nervous system, for overcoming anger and for strong character.

Keme

Day of the dead, who are stars, who are in space. We ask for good rest and for strength from the dead so the serenity and joy that reign in the essence of our lineage of having lived on Mother Earth may be ours. They guide and accompany us during our existence, helping avoid all kinds of danger. Usually, a ceremony is held in the cemetery for healing, physical, mental, and spiritual energy cleansing, and cleansing of envy or difficult obstacles in life.

Kej

Four cosmic points, destiny of humanity, feminine strength, agility. A day for asking for physical and spiritual strength, for being responsible with our actions and confident in ourselves. The energy of being supportive. A day to pray for a pregnancy.

Q'anil

Germination, life, creation. The energy of the human seed and the diversity of seeds about Mother Earth. The spirit of corn. On this day, a ceremony is held to thank and ask for a good harvest and everything Mother Earth gives us: food, animals, life, rain. A time to give thanks for the children and for their good growth, and for healing diseases of the skin and blood.

Toj

Symbolic offering to nature. The glue for life. A day to ask for good action for the prevention of emotional diseases, chronic and degenerative problems. A time to reflect on how, if our actions are positive, we will reap positive things, and if our actions are bad, the consequences are difficult because it is important to be in harmony with our environment and with ourselves.

Tz'i

Friendship, authority, fidelity. A day to ask for a good birth. It is the law of nature and human law, order and accuracy. On this day, a ceremony is held to resolve legal problems, and divine intervention to solve any type of illnesses and problem. A time for divine justice to arrive.

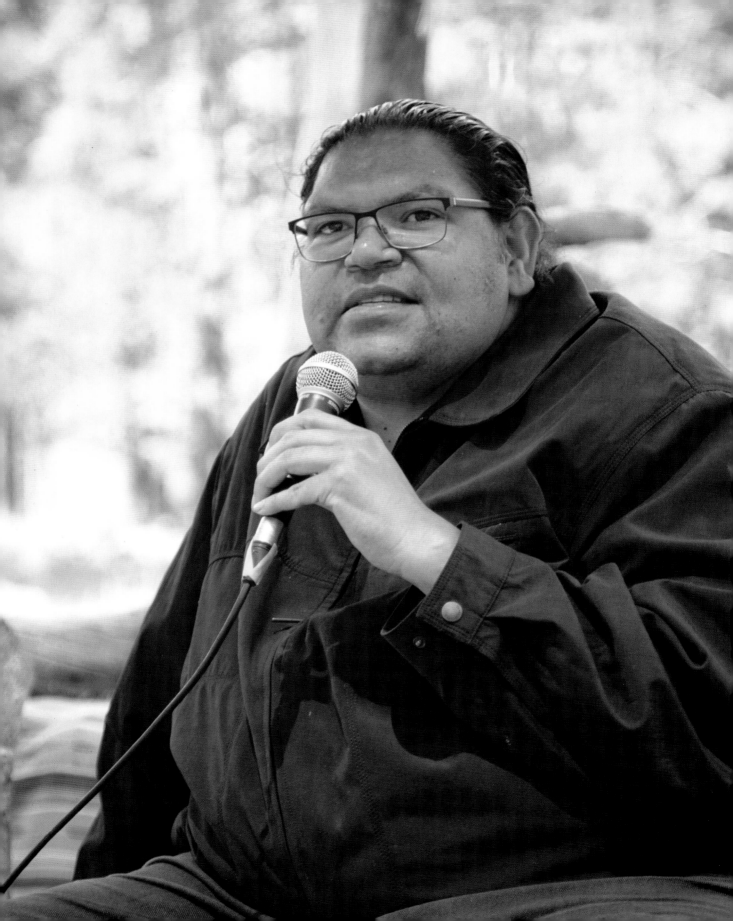

WARREN ROBERTS

Thunghutti and Bundjalung ✳ Australia

Warren Roberts is a proud Thunghutti and Bundjalung man focused on creating connection and unity between Aboriginal and Torres Strait Islander People and non-Indigenous Australians. He has been fortunate enough to work alongside esteemed Aboriginal and Torres Strait Islander elders, who have encouraged him to reflect on the importance of respecting cultural protocols. His focus is to empower Aboriginal and Torres Strait Islander People to build their capacity to be self-determining by organizing within the community, while also creating spaces in the broader Australian society through relationships with non-Indigenous communities and organizations (including government). Warren's community organizing is facilitated through the ancient cultural practices of storytelling and yarning, which he learned from his elders. He continues this tradition through his day-to-day life and YARN Australia, the organization he founded in 2007.

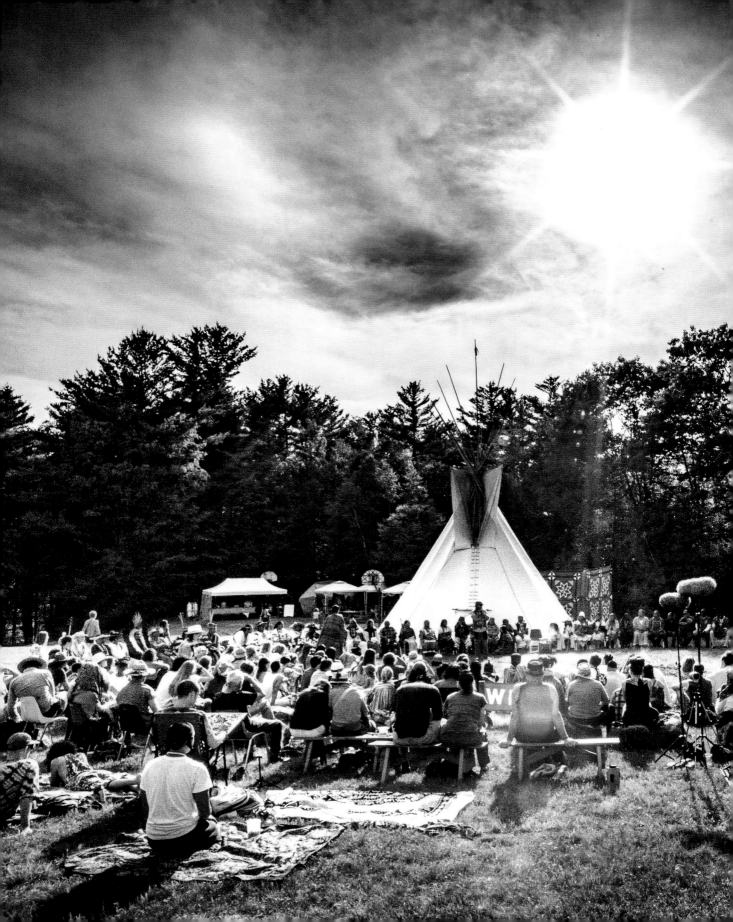

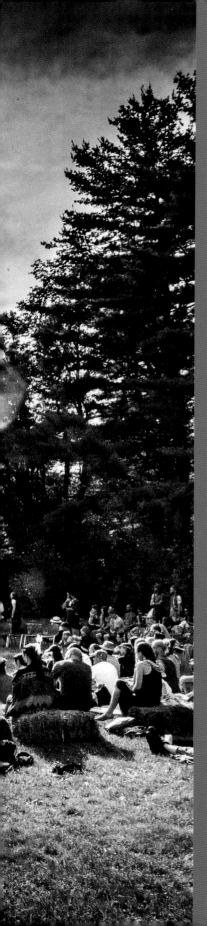

Ceremony
Tradition and Story

❋

Ceremony is sacred action. To initiate, to pass on, to carry the essence of life we have been given and must share is at the heart of every culture's ceremony call. Hear from the elders about what they have learned through the ceremonies that define their homes, how they listen and how they call in the passage of their culture's sacred songs.

———

Notice what and how the elders speak about ceremony through tradition and story.

Deep Listening

Warren Roberts
Thunghutti and Bundjalung ✳ Australia

*The original sovereign Nations of Australia
are storytelling cultures.*

Our ancestors have shared their knowledge across generations, passing on their worldview through stories. It is a great responsibility to continue this tradition, and I believe everyone should aspire to become a storyteller and to engage with this unique and meaningful way of being.

My name is Warren Roberts. My work has encouraged me to reflect on the importance of respecting cultural protocols and the wisdom of our traditions. I founded YARN Australia to create intentional relationships between the original sovereign Nations of Australia and all peoples of Mother Earth through storytelling.

I share these three stories with you to offer a reflection of my way of being. I believe that by sharing stories with one another, our collective trust strengthens and our relationships grow, inspiring greater consciousness in our lives and our communities.

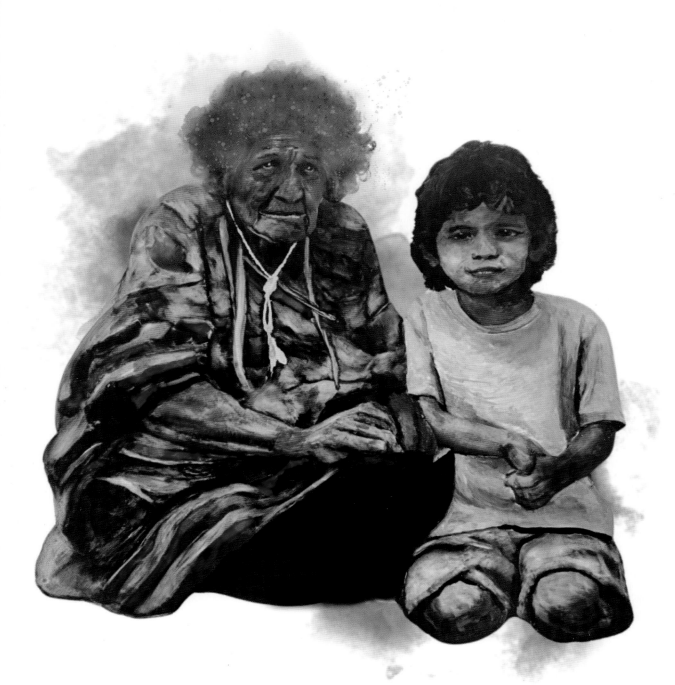

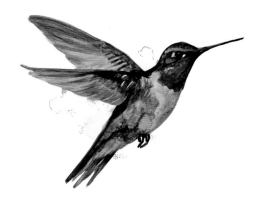

Deep Listening

On a warm sunny morning, sitting beside his grandpa, eating cereal on the deck outside his grandparents' wooden house, Nulla felt at home in Thunghutti Country. These were special moments, just the two of them together, the young boy and the old man, when no one could interrupt the quiet time they shared.

His grandpa turned to Nulla, gave him a gentle smile, and asked, "Can you hear that?" Nulla looked into his grandpa's big brown eyes, tilted his head to one side, and asked with interest, "What, Grandpa, do I hear what?" His grandpa raised his arm and swept it out, over the bush behind the house, "The wind, Nulla. Can you hear the wind?"

Nulla put down his spoon, looked up at his grandpa, and listened. Nulla then turned and looked at the eucalyptus trees nearby. He could hear the wind moving the branches, and as the tree branches swayed, they made a swishing sound, as though they were sighing. "Yes Grandpa," Nulla said excitedly, "I can hear the wind."

As he spoke, the wind strengthened and the air was full of sounds: chirrups of myna birds, the barking of a neighbor's dog, wind chimes tinkling from the house next door, the warbling song of a blackbird, and tutt-tutting of a noisy little mudlark. The old man smiled at his grandson, "The wind is full of sounds if you hear them, and if you really listen, you can hear more and more."

Together, they sat listening as the wind rose and fell, carrying sounds—voices, birds, traffic—that mixed with ease, with the cool breeze, creating a natural harmony. His grandpa had unlocked a secret for him. Nulla felt a warmth in his heart as he listened. He felt his connection to those natural sounds; he felt his place there in that moment, in his country, in his life.

Suddenly, the kookaburra laughed, loudly declaring his presence with his cheerful call. They had company. Grandpa and Nulla looked at each other and they laughed too.

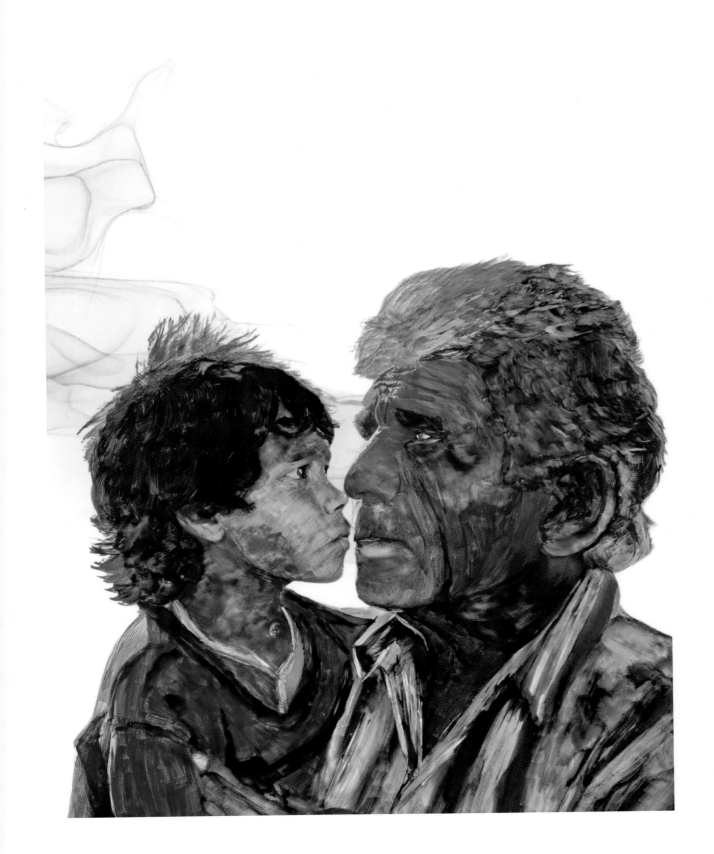

Intentional Storytelling

The morning light came through the curtains and Nulla opened his eyes. A warm feeling spread through him when he realized he was at his nanna's house. He liked staying at his grandparents' home; there were always fun things for him to do there, and he had all of their attention and could listen to the wisdom they shared with him.

Nulla jumped out of bed and raced into the kitchen. His nanna was at the bench with a big bowl preparing food as the whole family was coming over. Nulla asked his nanna, "What are you going to make?" She raised her eyebrows and responded, "Johnnycakes!" Nulla asked if he could help. "Of course, you can, Bub, but first you better have some breakfast."

Nulla ate some food, and, when he finished, he washed his hands so he could help his nanna cook. Nulla dragged a chair over to his nanna's side and climbed on top of it. Nanna tied a big apron around Nulla's tummy to keep his clothes clean and then rolled up his sleeves, so they would be clean too. Nulla watched as she poured in some flour, added a pinch of salt, cut some butter into the mixture, and, finally, added some water. She then went to the pantry and took out a jar, which she brought to the bowl and, with a spoon, added it to the mixture. Nulla asked Nanna, "What's that?" She responded, "It's my secret ingredient."

Nanna mixed the ingredients and her little helper helped. Nulla squeezed the flour and butter together—it was sticky—and the dough got stuck between his fingers. The flour would fly up into his face as he pummeled and stretched the mixture. Nanna laughed at his efforts, "It's alright, Bub, it's not a race." Nulla looked at his nanna, with flour in his eyebrows and in his black curly hair, and smiled a big smile. She smiled back and told him, "It's turning into dough."

Together, they made the balls of dough into johnnycakes, flattening them with their hands.

"How do we cook them, Nanna?" Nulla's tummy was rumbling.

Nanna took out the biggest frying pan from the cupboard and put it on the stove. She added butter to it, which melted with the heat. "Like this, Bub. When the butter melts and starts to hiss, we put in the johnnycakes and let them cook—first one side, then the next."

The air filled with the smell of butter and johnnycakes, and, when they were ready, Nanna put them on a big plate, with a spoonful of butter melting on top. The family arrived and the kitchen filled with cousins, aunties, and uncles. Nulla and his nanna served the johnnycakes with all kinds of toppings and kept on cooking them until they were all gone.

After a little rest, Nanna took Nulla and his cousins out for a walk, beyond the houses, in the bush. Nulla and his cousins walked in a line behind Nanna, through the long grass, toward some old trees. The scent of eucalyptus was strong in the air, and the sound of cicadas surrounded them. Nanna kept on walking and walking toward an old, old tree. "This is the one," she said, and she put her hand into a hollow branch. Nulla could see lots of little bees flying out, and when his nanna removed her hand, it was covered in bush honey. "Try some," she told Nulla and his cousins, and they all dipped their fingers into the golden pool in her hand. It was delicious, and the taste reminded Nulla of the johnnycakes. Suddenly, he remembered the mixture, "Hey, Nanna, is this your secret ingredient?" His Nanna shook her head with a big, beautiful smile, "What gives you that idea, Bub?"

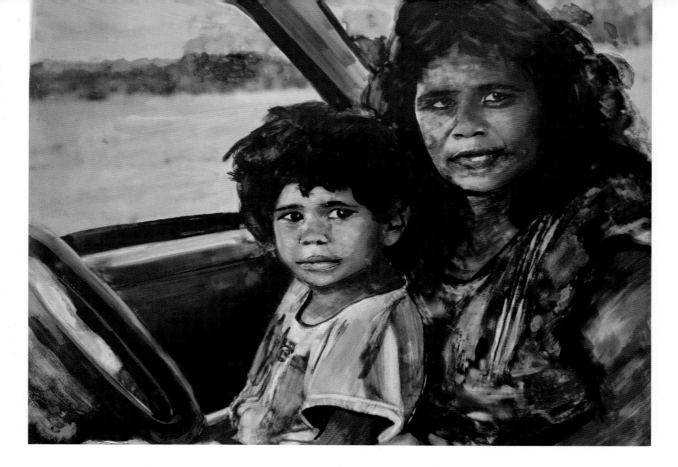

Time

It was time for Nulla to leave his grandparents' house. He was sitting in the back of his mum's car, as dust rose around them, and the car pulled slowly out of the long driveway. His nanna and grandpa stood waving until Nulla couldn't see them anymore, but he kept waving anyway; he felt sad he was leaving, but also full from his time with them.

Nulla looked out through the window at Thunghutti Country. He felt it was where he belonged, he knew it was where he belonged, where his family had always lived, under those stars at night, beside that river to fish, the place his family would always meet and be together. It was their place.

The road passed by the big gum trees and under the waratahs. Nulla wound down the window to catch the breeze and to see the country better. He could see a bush covered in wild strawberries, and he knew his nanna would pick them and make the berries into jam before the birds could eat them. It made him smile.

They passed a grass tree, which had berries too. He thought the magpies would enjoy them. He noticed so much more, having walked with his grandparents through the bush near their house, under the trees, beside the creek, and down to the river. He felt like his eyes had been opened in a new way. The car passed a massive bottlebrush covered in red blossoms, with lorikeets busy eating the honey, and he remembered the honey his nanna had found. So yummy.

Yes, he was sad to leave, but he knew he would be so welcome and delighted to return, to be comforted and refreshed by his country.

The Feagaiga (Sacred Promise or Covenant) with Mother Earth

Papali'i Dr. Tusi Avegalio
Polynesia ✳ Oceania

Our sense of kinship with our Mother Earth is in our language.

The very language of our people is rooted in the fact that we are born from the Earth.

Our umbilical cord is connected to the Earth. When I was born, my umbilical cord was cut and wrapped in ti leaves, and then buried in a secret location in my family's village. I had no idea what that meant. It wasn't until postgraduate school that I even thought to find out. So, what does it mean? Why do you bury your umbilical cord? Fortunately, my elder was still alive when I sought to ask why. It was a good time, because knowledge was actually outrunning wisdom. They were still alive so it gave me the opportunity to allow wisdom to catch up.

The reason, I was told, that my umbilical cord was wrapped in a ti leaf and then buried in the ground was to remind me my entire life that I have two mothers. My birth mother and, by the symbol of the burial of the umbilical cord, my Earth Mother. It was my responsibility to protect and defend them both—to see to their health, to see to their beauty, and to see to their

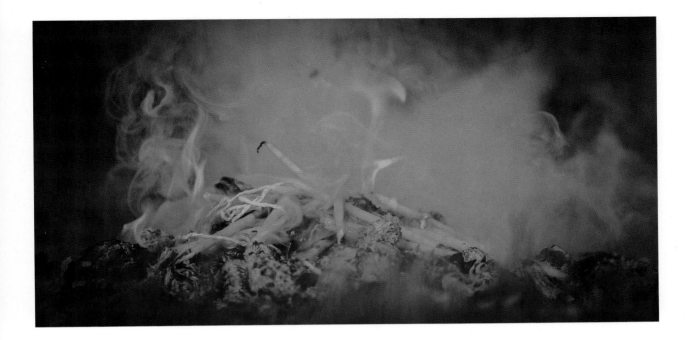

nourishment. It was only then that I began to realize why I have a level of comfort. When my biological mother passed away, I realized she's now with my Earth Mother. I look around me with all the trees and the birds and everything else. My mother's with them. When you have that kind of assurance, you're not easily attracted by material things.

As you get older, it's easier. You really understand there's a difference between being rich and being wealthy. There are a lot of people who are rich who are among the most miserable people I've ever met. The wealthy—they are incredible. They resonate. There's nothing that can provide greater richness, not only in your surroundings but within your own being, than being profoundly in love with those things you love most and who love you. For me, it's my grandchildren. My wife and my grandchildren. So, what is the greatest pleasure for me? When I can take their little hands and we walk around and we can look at an orchid, or the heliconia and pua. All the beautiful things. I can point to the sky and then I can take her to the beach. She can run around and play because I'll teach her that the Earth is the heart, but the ocean is the lungs of Moana (ocean); and by learning to swim and float, she's breathing with the lungs of Moana.

That's the kind of education to supplement STEM that is not being taught in schools. I think if we can weave the wisdom of the ancients with the science of the modern perspectives, especially quantum mechanics, I think we will be preparing our children and our leaders for a promising future.

The Feagaiga Covenant Ceremony

The wisdom passed down by our ancestors tells us that all humans have two mothers: our biological birth mother and our Earth Mother. In Polynesia, a newborn's umbilical cord is wrapped in ti leaves and ceremonially buried in the sacred ground. The physical act of the burial ceremonially conducted by elders symbolically connects the newborn to Papa, or Earth Mother.

Today, the modern meaning of "fanua" in Sāmoa is "land." Its original and ancient meaning is placenta or afterbirth. "'Ele'ele" means "dirt" and "palapala" is "mud." The original and ancient meaning of both words is blood. "Ma'a" means "stone," but its original meaning comes from the word "fatu ma'a," which means "heart." The very language of ancient Polynesia discerns the Earth as living and as the mother that birthed all life and material from the progenitor of the heavens, Tagaloa Lagi.

All elders of Polynesia are revered as the living stewards of the seeds of our living covenant to Papa, the Earth Mother. It is believed that the life tree within our elders bears and carries the seeds of the living covenant that is passed on to each generation by breathing it into every new life.

Holding the newborn, the grandmother or senior elder conducts a ceremonial prayer over the infant that ends by breathing into the child's nose and mouth. In that manner, the spiritual seeds of the covenant are planted within the child's lungs.

The mana, or spiritual energy carried by the breath of the elder, enters the child and flows throughout with the child's every breath carrying the seeds of the covenant to the extremities.

In time, the infant's body and covenant grow into a living oneness. The covenant and infant become one and the same. Hence, every child is and must be treated as a living covenant and a reminder to all of the promise between human and Earth Mother.

As a living covenant, it is the responsibility of all in the village to nurture and cultivate each child with alofa (love), until the fruits of maturity are expressed through actions of respect and love that reaffirm the covenant in all humans with Papa.

The basis of the covenant is the reaffirmation of love, respect, and actions that are consonant with the balance, beauty, harmony, health, sustainability, and wellness of Papa and Tagaloa's gifts of life to tagata māo'i (genuine or native human being in Sāmoan; the Hawaiian term "Kanaka Maoli" has an identical meaning.) It is the collective responsibility of all adults of the village (human society) to nurture and cultivate the health, well-being, and wellness of all children as repositories of the ancient promise.

The seeds of the covenant, when mature, produce the fruits of alofa (love) and fa'aaloalo (respect), which are the basis for harmony between humans and the universe, humans and nature, human and fellow human, and human and self. It is only when all four harmonies are consonant with each other that there is true balance, harmony, and peace on earth.

Papa's health, wellness, beauty, and life are dependent on the harvest of love and respect produced by the covenant.

With the symbolic connection created by the burial of the umbilical cord in the Earth, human fate is inextricably bound to the fate of Papa. If Papa is well, humans will be well. If Papa is ill, humans will become sick. If Papa is dying, humans will die.

The Chant of the Covenant

*The whales have lost their way . . . the sea tern that chooses one mate for life
flies alone . . . the coral is burned by the Sun . . .
the winds carry the salt of your tears.*

*All are reminders that we have misplaced our Feagaiga (covenant)
with our Mother Earth.*

*We have misplaced our Feagaiga by holding it aloft where the birds of
self-interest and pride have pecked on it; we have placed it upon the ground
where creatures of greed, profit, and exploitation have crawled over it; we have
held it in our trembling hands with timidity where it has hardened with the
mold of creatures that hide from the light of the sun.*

*We thank the great winds for reminding us that the Feagaiga (covenant)
is something that one does not hold up in the air,
lay upon the ground, or hold in one's hand;
that a Feagaiga's life is not possible outside of our own.*

*We will place our Feagaiga (covenant) between our hearts and our lungs so that
as long as our heart beats and our lungs breathe, our Feagaiga lives.*

*So long as we live, our covenant will live; so that we will see to your health,
your wellness, and your beauty.*

*We will help the whale find its way; the sea tern to find its mate, the waves to
comfort the coral, and the winds to carry the message of life.
Return to your dwellings, lands, and islands and breathe life in all
that you do; aloha (love), aloha, aloha oe.*

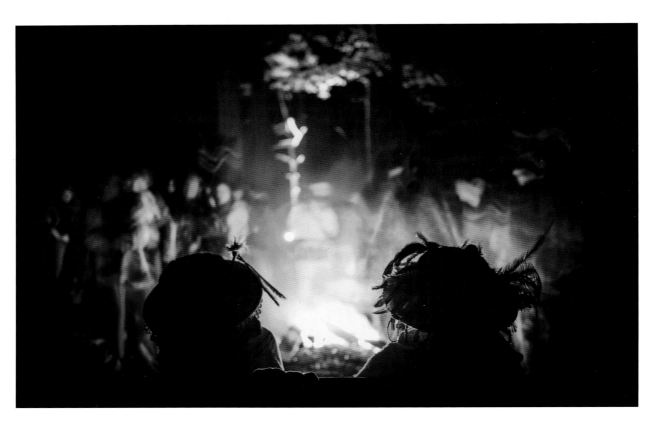

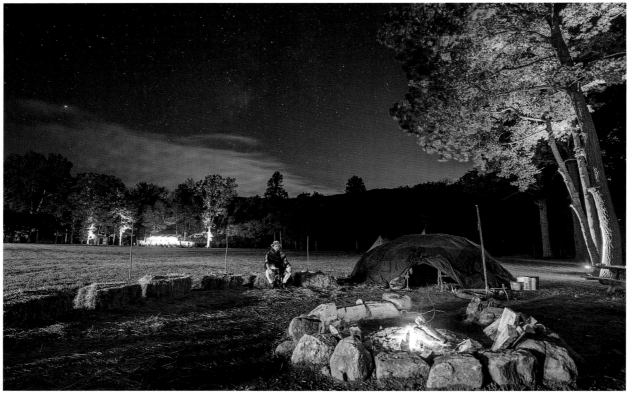

Connect with Your Ancestors

Grandmother Clara Soaring Hawk
Ramapough Lenape ❊ United States

It's important to understand who you are.

Anyone can remake themselves over and over. The truth of who you are, though, you can never run away from. For me, it seemed I was always out of place. I would always do things left when everyone did them right. I felt like I was living in the world, but I existed someplace else. I was able to find out what was going on with me by checking my ancestry. When you can visually see who your ancestors are, clarity arrives. It gives much meaning to the way I think—the way I raised my children, my need to be in the woods where I feel safest.

It's important for you to know your ancestry. When we're living today, we're living for the next seven generations. We will be the next ancestors. If it's not important to know your ancestors, what importance do you put on today in your life? Do you know what difference you could make in the next four, five, or six generations? I want someone I'm an ancestor of to feel like I'm worthy, that I've done something in this world that warrants staying remembered, that warrants calling me forth to continue to do good work. Our ancestors are still here and doing good work.

I have altars everywhere, like people, every place you can look. I call them "little stations." I have an altar for my mom, my father, and my youngest daughter who are my ancestors. I don't care how young they are with age. Once they transition, they're no longer here. They enter that world of supernatural knowledge. I set up a place where you can go and honor them.

For an altar, you might want to put up a picture, or something very special and personal that, perhaps, may have been given to you. It's always important to have candles, to have the light. I don't care how small the flame—when it's dark, that flame is seen so brightly. When you honor your ancestors in that way, just speak your heart. First, give thanks to Creator for where you are in your present place. Be thankful for all you have, for all you know, and that you've been called to serve.

We have to know our ancestors. Our ancestors stay with us. They protect us. They guide us. The more you are involved with knowing that your ancestors are present, the more present they are and the more you feel them. People might say it's crazy, but it's not. It's so real. The more you acknowledge their presence, the more they thank you. They say thank you for not forgetting about us, thank you for keeping us around, for allowing us to continue. It's not just the next seven generations we keep in our hearts, we give thanks to all the ancestors as well.

I think people come back as angels. We have angels all around us. If you had issues with someone who passed, you still have the opportunity and ability to fix that relationship. Once our relatives transition, that's all they want for us. No matter who is right or wrong, they want us to be okay, to have peace, to be able to move forward in a good way. When we have difficulties, even little things, maybe you misplace your keys, you can ask an angel to help you retrieve those keys. When you put this into practice, it is incredible—there's no more losing things! Whatever you need, there are angels all around who have been assigned to help us in every way.

Most of the angels around us in our lifetime will leave never having an assignment. All the years they've been assigned to you, all they ever wanted was to be useful. They're the worker angels. They need to work. I hear them saying, "I'm a worker. Put me on assignment. Give me something to do." This is all they're here for. That's how they live. That's how they thrive. We don't use them. We try to do it ourselves. We don't have to do everything ourselves. They are here, and they will help.

At the altar, give thanks for everything you are, for everything you have. Speak whatever you're thankful for that comes to your heart. Know that without your ancestors, none of it would have been possible. None of it. Know that you're being guided, and, if there's a teaching moment, they will come forth to help you learn. Give gifts like a plate of food, lighting a candle, tobacco, or burning sweetgrass. Even your words can be a gift.

I grew up in a big family and very few people know that fact. Most would think I was an only child, but that is because I was raised by my ancestors. I've had visions and dreams my whole life. Always speaking with someone and listening to someone you know is there, but nobody else can see. Know how real your ancestors are. Know they are here. The ancestors are as real and present as we are. That's how you should speak to them when you pray.

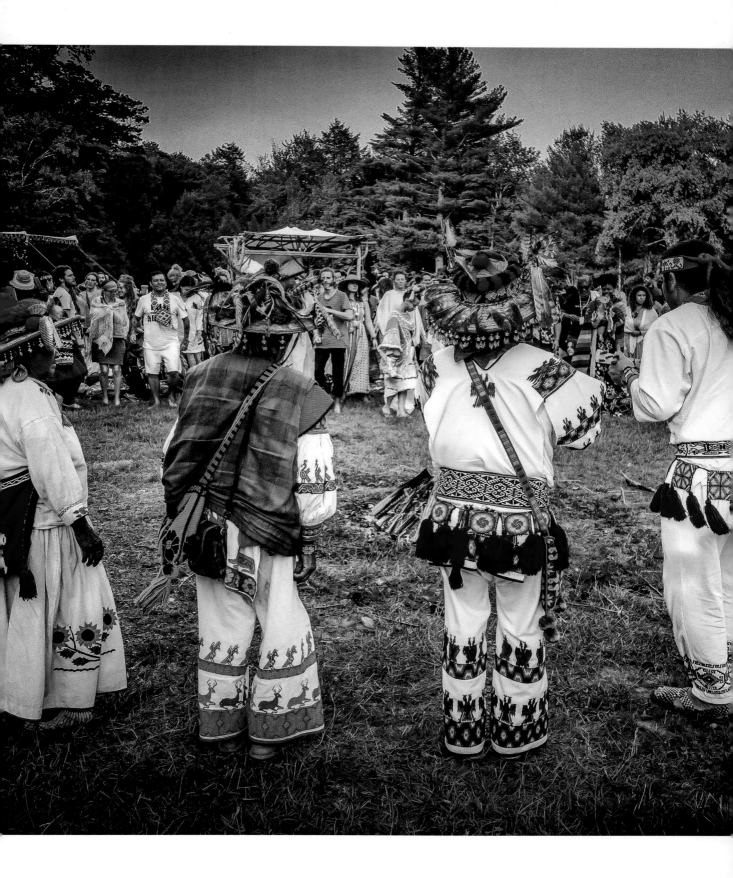

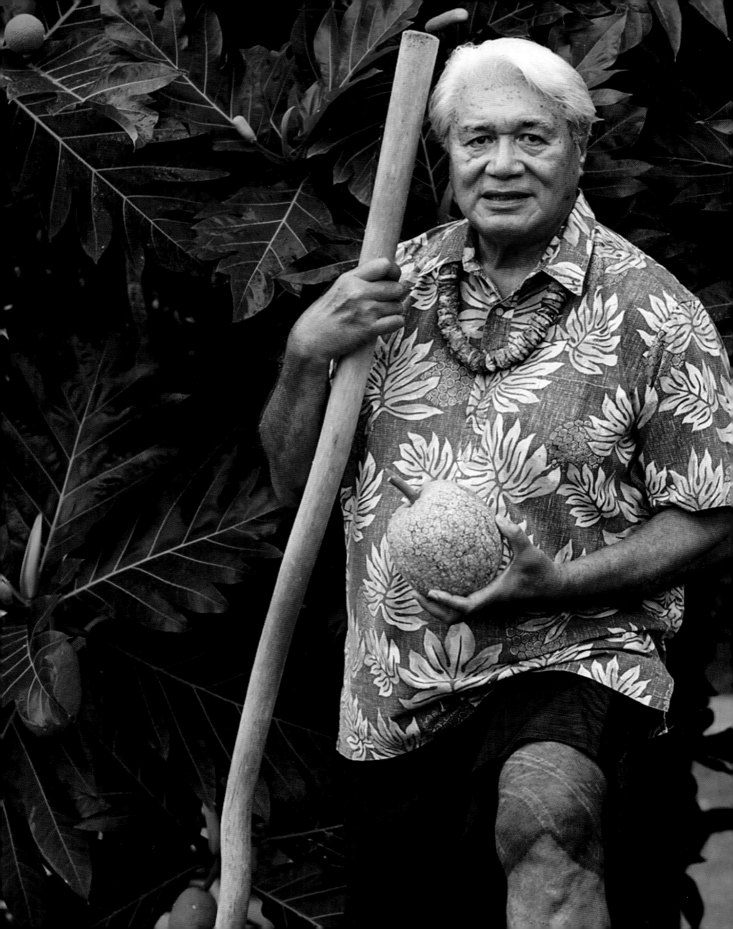

PAPALI'I DR. TUSI AVEGALIO

Polynesia ✤ Oceania

Papali'i is a Polynesian traditional leader from the Sāmoan Islands with extensive genealogical ties throughout the island cultures of Micronesia, Melanesia, and Polynesia, and he is a culturally based regenerative development advocate of Oceania. He promotes the weave of traditional wisdom, cultural values, and spiritualism with modern science, knowledge, and technology. He is also a Suli Matua (senior heir) to the Sa Malietoa Talavou warrior king line of Sāmoa and was conferred the Papali'i title in 1980 recognizing him as such.

Papali'i was raised in a social-cultural and spiritual context that views the Earth as his Earth Mother, accentuated by the ceremonial burial of his umbilical cord wrapped in lau ti leaves into the sacred ground as an infant. His i'ike (ability to attune to the rhymes, patterns, and currents of mana) aligns with the wisdoms of regeneration, symbiosis, and synergy inherited from his open ocean-voyaging ancestors. He cherishes the wisdom of his ancestor, Salamasina, the last and only queen of the Sāmoan Islands. Though an heir of a warrior line, the wisdoms of Salamasina have reframed the values of conquest and war to tofas (wisdoms) and healing that guide the definition of leadership to this day.

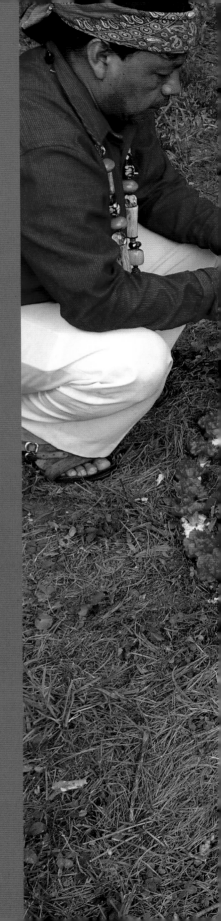

Love

Forgiving

✳

Love is what holds us together. Hear from the elders about how to live with the energy of love to bring us closer and to strengthen the bonds that uphold our global home.

Notice what and how the elders speak about love through forgiving.

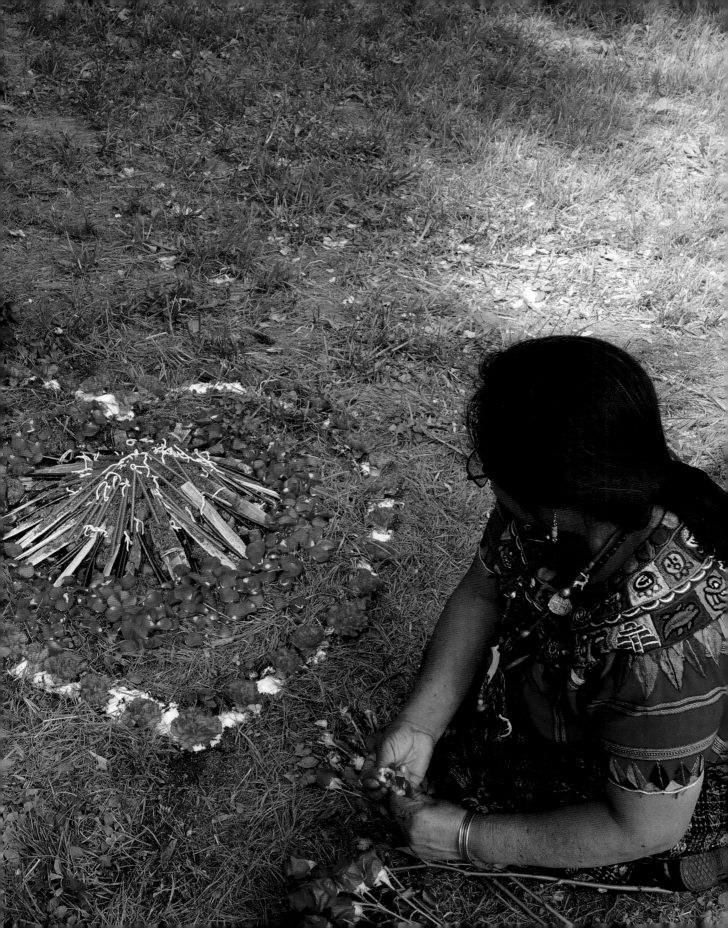

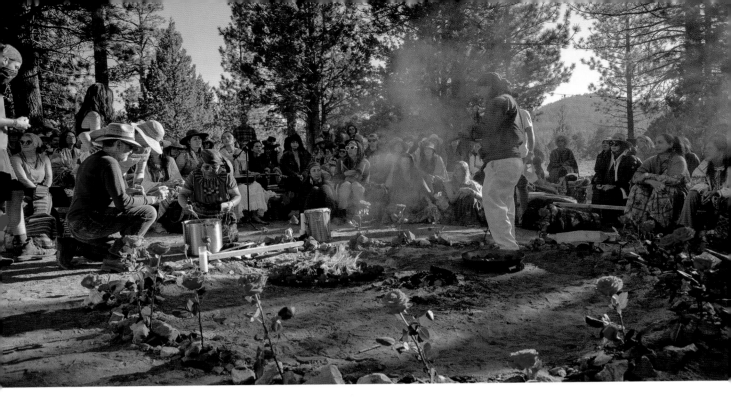

Bring in Love

Nana Amalia Tum Xinico

Maya Kaqchiquel ☀ Guatemala

People suffer so much if they can't find a partner.

The first thing I do for people when they come to me is clear the way to make them see the attitude and help people see love for themselves first. They have to have enough love for themselves. If a person loves themself, cares for themself, cuddles, hugs, and gives themself flowers, there is no need for someone else to give them a bouquet of flowers. They, themselves, can flourish within themselves.

Sometimes, when people need this love for themselves, they cannot see love. They only wait for someone's love to love them, to cuddle them, to let the flowers come, to let the compliments come; but they are very hard on themselves. So, first is acceptance. Love for oneself. Then, it is valid to ask the energies.

Put a red candle down. This is the symbol of love for you. Write down your name on a piece of paper. Place it below the candle and give all your requests. It is recognizing yourself. Who you are. Are you angry? Are you happy? Are you harmonious with yourself?

Ask the great universe, Mother Earth, the Nahuals, the energies, the Great Creator, maker of life to open that path: "Let that person come to me."

The right person. The person who really respects you. The person who really loves you, without conditions . . . that is what you are requesting.

Give a flower. When I say give a flower, I mean to make your altar, put a photograph there on your altar, put a glass of water, your flower, and it is for who you are. You are the person you are worshiping. Give yourself a hug. What are you giving to this body? What are you giving to this stomach? What thoughts are you putting in your head? What feelings are you giving to your heart?

Write down all your feelings, all your emotions on a piece of paper. Do this in one ceremony, not every day. What are the things you no longer want to have? What are the thoughts that should no longer be there, that do not belong to you? If there are also issues that you have been generating from your family lineage, simply say, "Thank you, Mom; thank you, Dad; thank you brother. Thank you ancestors, but, today, I want to make my life. Today, I want all that does not correspond to me to be cut."

Then, you can do what belongs to you.

Do what you feel in your heart. You can burn the paper. Find a river, blow on the paper three times, and leave it in the river. The river teaches us. The river never returns. The water flows even though there are so many stones, even though there are so many stumbles. Water always finds its way and flows. The human being must learn from water to flow and not stay stuck with the feelings that exist. Throw away all those thoughts that no longer serve you.

You have to believe in the ceremony you are doing to begin to change, little by little, your attitude, your lifestyle, your thoughts, to release, and so find your loved one on your path.

Love, not just love as a couple, is self-love. Love to everything. Self-love is knowing what your energy is. All your essence is concentrated there.

Find out what your energy is from your Nahual Maya and be attentive for the day to do that energy because that's when your whole being is born.

Through your Nahual comes all your intelligence, all your personality—and also all your weaknesses. You can look it up online with your date of birth.

Love energy is the thread of life. To begin to weave that love, I recommend people use two red candles. Then, make two hearts for this person to come and ask the great universe for them to appear in the space where you are, between friendships or at your place of work. The right person can be anywhere. Sometimes people are shy. They don't like to talk and they don't have friends.

The energy through the two candles opens the way. It doesn't need to be a big ceremony. The symbol of a couple, the symbol of duality, is simply asking the great Creator of life, father, mother, space, Earth to send love your way.

Use red flowers, like roses or carnations. Draw a heart on the ground with the flowers or with sugar (white, red, or pink). What we want is sweetness. It can be made with honey too.

Place the two red candles in the middle of the heart and ask that the path for romantic love and partnership is opened.

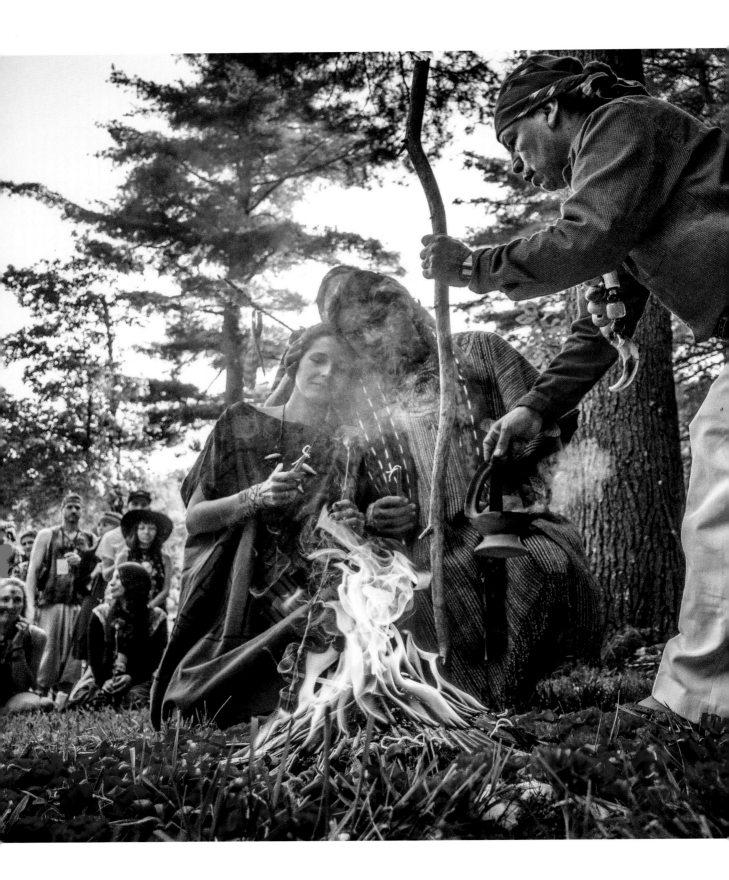

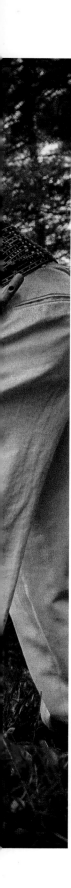

Forgiveness

Papali'i Dr. Tusi Avegalio

Polynesia ✻ Oceania

The ancients knew we live in a universe suffused
with the omniscient.

Knowing all over. An omniscient presence that many traditions and religions call "spirit." What is fascinating is that modern quantum physics confirms it is energy. In Polynesian, we call it "mana"—the breath of life from our Earth Mother. In many of the islands, she's called Papahānaumoku. On all the islands, she's known as Moana, the Polynesian name for the Pacific Ocean and Earth Mother in general. Complementing the breath of life is the heaven father of the Polynesians, Tagaloa Lagi. The entity, the essence that is omnipresent, that is all over. Moana and Tagaloa Lagi. They breathe the spirit, the breath of life. It goes into the lungs of our elders. They, in turn, breathe it into our children.

It is the children who are the custodians of mana in its purest form. Then, mana matures in their lives as they get older and, eventually, they release it. Hence, the child and the elder are fundamental to the breath of life. They are our sacred trust. We have a belief:

- ✖ If you want to be a good leader, remember to make sure that knowledge can enable and assure that our children are well fed and healthy.

- ✖ When you come back with knowledge, be sure to see that your elders are cared for with love and respect—that you can protect and defend.

- ✖ Assure that our women and our mothers live without fear.

- ✖ Make sure you can embrace and respect the sacredness of our kinship with Earth Mother.

Those are the four wisdoms the elders imparted to me as I left for university. I've now returned and retired. They have all passed on, but those lessons are central to my life and purpose.

Mana, the elders said, is everything. It includes the mighty whales, the giant redwood cedar trees, the tiny protozoa in water, air, land, fire, and ice. It includes everything. The creatures that swim or crawl or walk or fly, the four-legged and the two-legged, the visible universe and all that is hidden. All our spirit bound or unbound. Mana is divine energy and spirit is larger than the universe. It includes and interpenetrates everything.

So, there are many ceremonies and chants and protocols. All societies have them. Ceremonies celebrate life, birth, death, the beginning of a journey, aloha, healing, and forgiveness among many others. Of the many ceremonies that will be shared at some time, today I want to share a ceremony of healing unique to Sāmoa of the Polynesian Islands of the great Moana. It is called ifoga. It literally means to give, to offer, to present. Let me provide a context.

There was an actual situation in which an individual had gotten into an argument and killed a person from another village. In Sāmoa, as in many islands of Polynesia, there is no such thing as an individual. There is only family. So, when you harm one, you harm all. That is why Sāmoans are so proud and will basically stand at the drop of a dime when there is a sense of being offended or if they sense the need to protect and defend those things that are sacred to us—our children, our elders, our women, and our environment.

So, this individual killed this man who happens to be the son of the chief of a neighboring village. The elders of the perpetrator of the murder, once they understood, gathered together and knew that if this situation was not addressed immediately, guided by wisdom, blood would flow. Many innocent people would see devastation, and the destruction of land would be great. So, the elders got together, brought the perpetrator before them, and then spoke among each other, and said, "To whom do you place the greatest sacred love and respect and reverence?"

The perpetrator, in tremendous remorse and weeping, said it was his grandmother. The grandmother, being present and understanding the essence of ifoga, willingly stood up and said she would be remiss if she did not present herself in this manner.

She understood that mana, or aloha, is the only energy that can mitigate or soften the energy of anger and hate and revenge. Our ancients understood that you cannot destroy heat or negative anger. You cannot. The best you can hope for is you might be able to contain it, but it is not containable. They understood you cannot destroy hate, but you can transform it.

It's incredible the wisdom in how they were able to get it so, instead of preparing for war to support the wrong of one of their own, they prepared for love.

The grandmother, knowing her role was because of ifoga, and it was only through ifoga, through deep love, that healing is not only possible, but enduring.

The next stage, the village gets together and, led by the chiefs, they journey to the neighboring village. Of course, the village chiefs are alerted that there is a group coming from the village of the individual who killed one of their own. Because they saw the procession was a procession of family, there were no signs of weapons or war-like intentions, the village gathered as the procession entered the victim's village square.

They went before the great dwelling of the high chief and they all sat on the floor, on the ground, with the old lady seated in front before them. Then, a fine mat was draped over her head. The village sat there with their heads bowed and in deep mourning. The ceremony meant that the aggrieved, the father of the son who was murdered, can pick up his war club, walk down to where the grandmother was seated with the fine mat draped over her head, and slaughter her. Take her life in retribution for the life taken from his family. If that had occurred, the family would then wrap the body in the fine mat and carry her home ceremonially. All revenge, all purposes of restoration for balance and harmony, have been restored and it ends there. It never ends there, but at least ceremonially there will be no open acts of violence. People will see that the old lady had offered her life for peace and harmony with love. It would be shameful for anyone to violate her sacred aloha by engaging in any form or act of retribution, any act of violence, because it would be disrespectful for the spirit.

This is how we teach our young. This is one scenario.

The other scenario is that the chief can then pick up his war club and set it back down again. Then, he can walk to the old lady draped with the fine mat, remove the fine mat from her head, and bring her into his dwelling and immediately order food and drink and welcome her into his home. With that action, the village jumps up and prepares food and drink. They come out to the family of the old lady sitting in the village square, out into the hot sun, and bring food and drink to them. That is an act of forgiveness. By offering that which is the most sacred in return. The act of love is so moving and so powerful that forgiveness immediately begins. Healing. From then on, because of the elder's example of embracing the wisdom of the ages and understanding the power, by forgiving, healing occurs. The essence was aloha.

Now, what happened to the culprit? He will have to carry that for the rest of his life. He alone has to suffer what he saw, what he experienced, and then he will have to just deal with it, if he can. It is not unusual that such an individual is so shamed and so profoundly affected that they're never seen again.

The ifoga ceremony is an example through our history of our acts of love that have to be led by our leaders. You cannot expect it from a child. You cannot just talk about it by pulling a book off the shelf. You need to live it. You need to be the example.

Good leaders lead. Great leaders heal.

We should always strive as examples in the process of sharing and shaping great leaders who emerge from our families, from our societies, and from our world. Do small things with great aloha. If you cannot do things with great aloha. Do it with small aloha. The aloha grows when you serve.

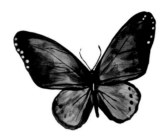

Braiding the Hair

Grandmother Clara Soaring Hawk and Grandmother Mona Polacca
Ramapough Lenape and Hopi, Havasupai, Tewa ⁑ United States

People don't realize braiding hair is very sacred.
It's almost a ceremony.

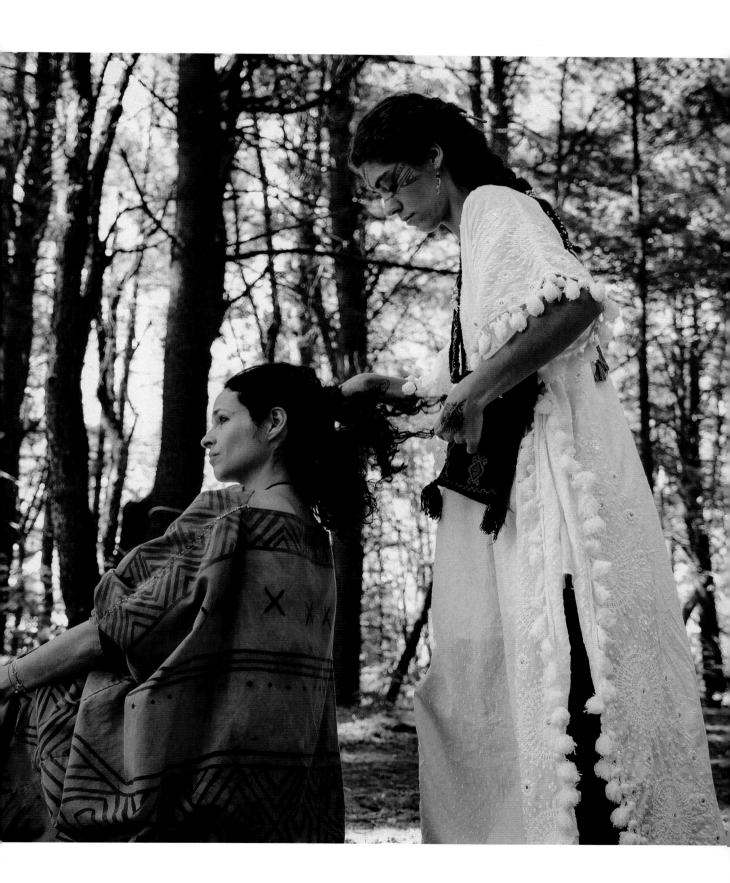

Grandmother Clara Soaring Hawk

Women will brush each other's hair. You don't just let anyone brush your hair, you know. What you're doing is allowing yourself to be vulnerable. You're sitting in front of someone who has access to you completely. They're behind you.

You see, a lot of natives have long hair. Even the men might have a long braid going down their back. That's the connection of your spinal column to your brain; the way it hangs from your head and lies down your back, the look of the braid is spine-like. The braid has both spiritual and physical significance to protect that connection between the spine and your brain.

Sweetgrass is the representation of Earth Mother's hair. That's one reason we braid it . . . like we braid our hair. I have a relationship with sweetgrass. I'm growing it. It looks beautiful. I talk to it. It's for us. It smells so sweet. It helps bring people together. When I make a friend, I say, "I have a feeling we'll be braiding sweetgrass together."

Growing up, someone would hold one end of the sweetgrass and the other person would braid it because, to get a good braid, you have to keep it tight. You have to have someone pulling on it just a bit. So it brings connection. It helps build the relationship in a good way.

It's good to give someone a sweetgrass braid when they're traveling because it carries good energy for safe travels. It carries sweet energy. We don't burn sweetgrass before we burn sage because sweetgrass invokes all energy. We burn sage first because it creates a safe space. Sweetgrass, then, invites, pulls in the ancestors.

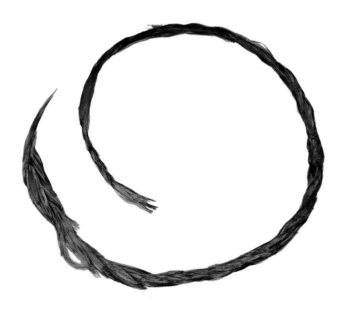

Grandmother Mona Polacca

When I was a child, part of my upbringing was the care for our hair. Not only my mother, but my aunties and my older sisters as well as my extended family, sisters, and cousins. We all took care of each other's hair.

I always remember how they would bathe us and wash our hair. Our hair was always allowed to grow. It wasn't cut. Our hair grew out and grew long. As we were growing up, we would always fix our hair into little braids. I used to do this with my daughter, even though the hair was still really fine and really short. I remember a time as a child when I had just woken up. I came out and my hair was blown everywhere. My older brother looked at me and laughed. "What happened?" he asked. "Did you have a storm in your room last night?" So then, you know . . . I gotta fix my hair!

In our tradition, in fixing the hair you have, you're stimulating not only the hair and the roots, but also the mind or the brain. You're stimulating that through the touching of the head. How you comb it, how you pull it, how you braid it. Usually, the braids are three strands. That is the mind, the heart, and the body. It is a teaching of discipline. When someone is working on your hair, the discipline is that you sit still and you are present with whatever is with the movement of your hair. It stimulates your mind, your brain. It's such a relaxing feeling. It's like having your head massaged. It creates a sense of peacefulness. That calm comes over you. So you're there, you're present, and you're just experiencing your own body, mind, heart, all of that as one.

That's how we work with our children, our babies, as they're growing. We work on their hair. Among us, the hair isn't just grown long among the girls. The boys also grow their hair and take care of it that way too. By braiding the hair, it creates a sense of groundedness. There's energy in the air. It's like static energy, static electricity in the air. Usually, I feel it when it's windy. When the wind is blowing and it's blowing my hair around, I get that static electricity and my hair starts standing up like feelers or antennae floating around. It feels chaotic, to me anyway. I feel like there's this energy, this electricity going through me, which creates discomfort and, in some ways, affects the mood. When a child is fussy, crying, biting, just having a bad time, fix the hair. It keeps that child grounded. When there's static electricity and sometimes other things going on around them, that creates anxiety.

We say your hair is your mind. We're very careful about who we let touch our hair. We don't want anyone to come along and pull our hair. That's a violation. If someone you know pulls your hair, it's not acceptable. That's also partly why we braid the hair and keep the hair tied. It's helpful in managing where your hair goes, who touches your hair, and how your hair is being treated.

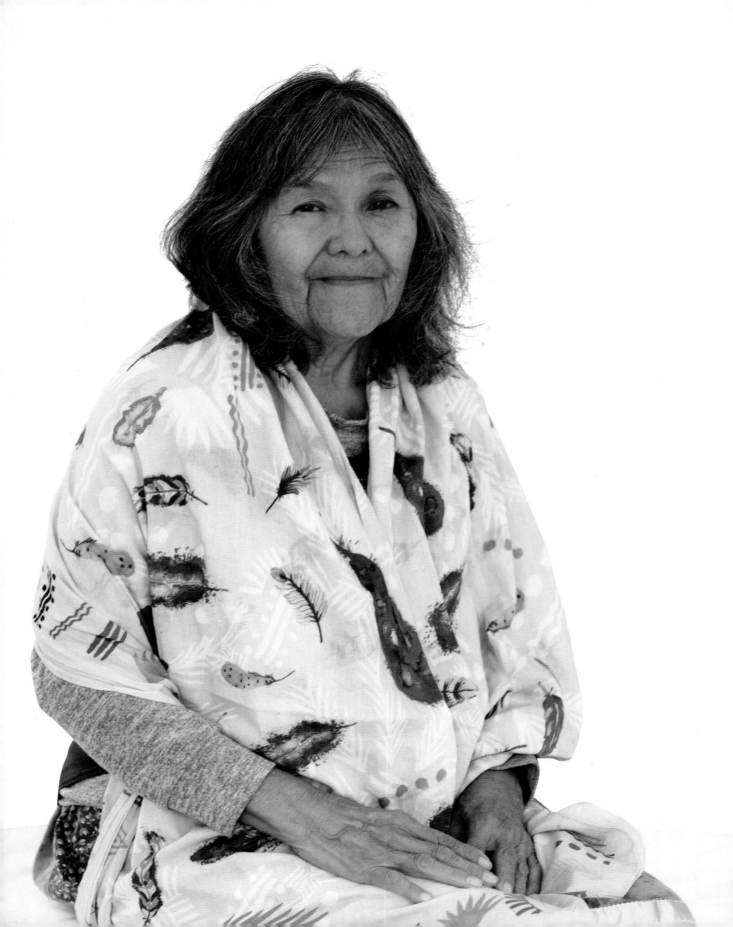

GRANDMOTHER MONA POLACCA

Hopi, Havasupai, Tewa ✳ United States

Mona is a Hopi, Havasupai, and Tewa Native American spiritual elder and water protector from Arizona. She has worked to further social justice for Indigenous People from an early age. She is an author in the field of social sciences, has held posts of responsibility as treasurer for her tribe, has served on several committees for Indigenous Peoples within the United Nations, and is widely known for her leadership in the Native American revitalization movement.

Mona has gained international recognition for her work as a founding member of the International Council of Thirteen Indigenous Grandmothers, a group of spiritual elders, medicine women, and wisdom keepers founded in 2004.

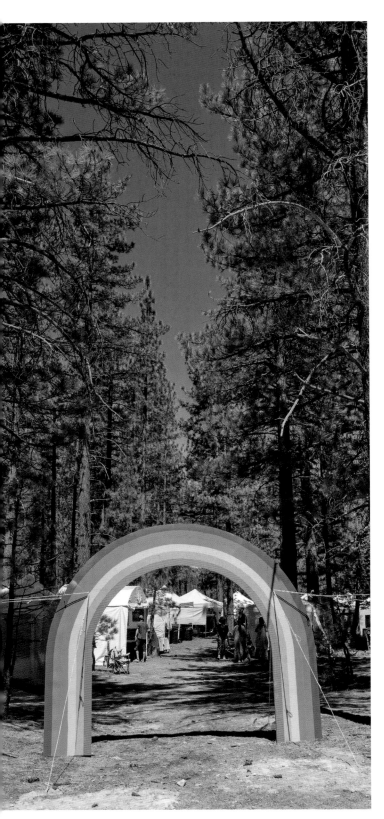

About Aniwa

Aniwa's Council of Elders includes some of the world's most renowned Indigenous Wisdom Keepers.

Our mission is to amplify the voices of Indigenous leaders, to help us remember how to connect with the power of the elements, the memories of the trees, the teachings of the heart. Together, we awaken and join forces in these times of great change.

Aniwa is a convergence of cultures and wisdom. Through immersive gatherings, retreats, and an online platform, we honor and preserve ancestral wisdom, promoting healing and environmental stewardship. We cultivate a deeper understanding of our shared mission as humanity, striving to inspire a collective commitment to living in harmony with nature and each other, ensuring that the timeless wisdom of Indigenous peoples continues to guide future generations.

www.aniwa.co

Acknowledgment

This book, *Sacred Ceremony for a Sacred Earth*, is a testament to the priceless wisdom shared with us by Indigenous elders from around the world. First and foremost, we extend our deepest gratitude to the elders and wisdom keepers who entrusted us with the teachings of their people. Their sacred ceremonies and traditions are the heartbeat of Aniwa, and we honor them and their lineages for carrying forward the ancient ways of healing and connection.

To the ancestors of these traditions, whose voices echo through the teachings within these pages, we offer our humble thanks. Your legacy lives on, not only through your descendants but through all who practice these sacred rituals with reverence: Apache, Diné, Hopi, Havasupai, Tewa, Inka, Paq'o Andino, Kaumatua (Maori), Maya Kaqchiquel, Maya K'iche, Polynesian, Ramapough Lenape, Thunghutti, Bundjalung, Wiwa, and Yoeme.

To the communities and families of the elders: Thank you for sharing your leaders with us. We recognize the deep responsibility that comes with carrying this wisdom and are committed to safeguarding and amplifying it with the utmost respect.

To our Aniwa Team, especially our visionary founder and CEO, Vivien Vilela: Your unwavering dedication, determination, passion, and spirit have supported this prayer to be manifested into reality.

To our COO, Elizabeth Garard: Your thoughtful and kind leadership has helped Aniwa blossom.

To our Aniwangels: Shantteh Petrossian, thank you for your commitment, tireless work, and all the sacrifices you have made to sustain this mission; Nikka Kurland, thank you for being a ray of sunshine, for your devotion to the elders, and for always taking such good care of them.

A special acknowledgement goes to Will Cady, whose skill in transcribing the elders' wisdom and weaving their words into a compelling narrative has brought this book to life. Your work ensures that the teachings' depth and spirit resonate throughout every page.

Thank you to Jill Alexander, our editor, and the team at The Quarto Group for approaching us for this book and their commitment to crafting this project.

Your respectful and thoughtful engagement has been essential in bringing these teachings to a wider audience with care and integrity.

We are immensely grateful to our friends and family who have supported us from the very beginning: Rudy Randa, Oscar Matzuwa, Melissa and Carlo Zola, Oona Chaplin and Anka Amaru, Jo Little and Mickey Curbishley, Kirsten and Matt Bigliardi, Dan Gieber, Ginny Griego, and Lena and Ahmed Agrama.

To the countless people who have participated in, supported, donated to, and volunteered at our Gatherings and initiatives—we are deeply grateful. Special thanks to Victoria Keon-Cohen, our Gathering producer, and Mitch Kirsh, our Gathering advisor, whose generous contributions have been invaluable.

To Ty Comfort for your generosity over the years and for making the very first Gathering possible.

Thank you to our 501(c)(3) organization, the Huya Aniwa Foundation and our trustee Laura Patterson for their efforts to preserve sacred lands and culture. We deeply appreciate your pivotal role in strengthening the Aniwa mission.

Our gratitude extends to the photographers and artists who capture the essence of Aniwa Gathering for this book.

◆ Photographers: Angela Farmer, Anura Elizabeth, Bryan Mir, Chris Dodds, Daniel Garcia, Erin Donalson, Ivan Sawyer Garcia, Jethro Tanner, Katya Castillo, Kelly Daniels, Marc Baptiste, Raine Skye, Ru, Safaa Kagan, and Ursula Vari

◆ Artists: Chiffon Lark and Eugene Baatsoslanii Joe

Lastly, to the future generations: May these sacred ceremonies continue to live through you, guiding you on the path of healing, unity, and reciprocity with all of Creation. Thank you for inspiring us to strive for a more beautiful tomorrow: Anhinga, Atzin, Amadeo, Atlantis, Camellia, Carmen, Everest, Gabriel, Lune, Marli, Ocean, River, Ronny, Siany, Sebastian, Tayo, and Teya.

With deepest respect and gratitude,
The Aniwa Co. Team

Index